Traditional Chinese Treatment for Otolaryngologic Diseases

Chief - Editor: Hou Jinglun
Editor: Zhao Xin, Li Guohua

Academy Press [Xue Yuan]

First Edition 1997
ISBN7 – 5077 – 1362 – 8

Traditional Chinese Treatment for Otolaryngologic Diseases
Chief – Editor: Hou Jinglun
Editor: Zhao Xin   Li Guohua

Published by
Academy Press [Xue Yuan]
11 Wanshoulu Xijie, Beijing 100036, China

Distributed by
China International Book Trading Corporation
35 Chegongzhuang Xilu, Beijing 100044, China
P. O. Box 399, Beijing, China

Printed in the People's Republic of China

Preface

Traditional Chinese Medicine and Pharmacology(TCMP) has a long history. It summed up abundant clinical experience in the struggle against diseases. It has formed an integrated, unique and first of all, a scientific system of both theory and clinical practice. On the fundamental principle of 'Zhengtiguannian'(Wholism) and 'Bianzhenglunzhi' (Treatment of the same disease with different therapies). TCM treatment is effective for various kinds of diseases with few side – effect taken. At present, a great upsurge in learning, practising and studying TCM is just in the ascendant. For the benefit of people of all countries, we compiled this series of 'Collections of Traditional Chinese Medicine' in order to promote the spread of TCM all over the world.

In this book, we introduced comprehensively TCM treatment for commonly encountered otolaryngologic diseases and therapies such as drug therapy, acupuncture and moxibustion, Qigong, massage, dietic therapy, etc. are suggested accordingly. This series is the best for those foreign friends who want to learn and master traditional Chinese medicine.

May everyone of all nations enjoy a healthy life!

Chief – Editor

Contents

Part One   Nasal Diseases

Chapter One	Acute Rhinitis	(1)
Chapter Two	Chronic Rhinitis	(5)
Chapter Three	Allergic Rhinitis	(11)
Chapter Four	Rhinitis Sicca	(17)
Chapter Five	Atrophic Rhinitis	(20)
Chapter Six	Acute Nasosinusitis	(26)
Chapter Seven	Chronic Nasosinusitis	(32)
Chapter Eight	Epistaxis	(38)
Chapter Nine	Nasal Vestibulitis	(47)
Chapter Ten	Rhinopharyngitis	(50)
Chapter Eleven	Nasal Furuncle	(53)
Chapter Twelve	Peripheral Facial Paralysis	(57)
Chapter Thirteen	Trigeminal Neuralgia	(66)

Part Two   Laryngopharyngeal Diseases

Chapter One	Acute Pharyngitis	(71)
Chapter Two	Chronic Pharyngitis	(76)
Chapter Three	Chronic Hypertrophic Pharyngitis	(82)
Chapter Four	Atrophic Pharyngitis	(84)
Chapter Five	Submucous Hematoma of Pharynx	(86)
Chapter Six	Acute Epiglottitis	(88)
Chapter Seven	Acute Tonsillitis	(92)
Chapter Eight	Peritonsillar Abscess	(97)
Chapter Nine	Pharyngeal Paraesthesia	(101)
Chapter Ten	Acute Laryngitis	(103)
Chapter Eleven	Acute Subglottic Laryngitis	(108)
Chapter Twelve	Chronic Laryngitis	(111)
Chapter Thirteen	Chronic Hypertrophic Laryngitis	(116)
Chapter Fourteen	Atrophic Laryngitis	(119)

Chapter Fifteen	Rhythmic Palatopharyngolaryngeal Muscular Clonus	(123)
Chapter Sixteen	Polyp of the Vocal Cord	(126)
Chapter Seventeen	Vocal Nodules	(130)
Chapter Eighteen	Vocal Edema	(133)
Chapter Nineteen	Vocal Mucosal Hemorrhage	(136)
Chapter Twenty	Cricoarytenoid Arthritis	(139)

Part Three   Aural Diseases

Chapter One	Acute Catarrhal Otitis Media	(143)
Chapter Two	Chronic Catarrhal Otitis Media	(149)
Chapter Three	Acute Suppurative Otitis Media	(152)
Chapter Four	Sudden Deafness	(157)
Chapter Five	Senile Tinnitus	(160)
Chapter Six	Nervous Tinnitus	(163)
Chapter Seven	Ménière's Disease	(167)

Part Four   Commonly Used Recipes

Decoction of Cinnamomi, Glycyrrhizae, etc.	(173)
Decoction of Cinnamomi, Paeoniae and Aemarrhenae	(174)
Antipyretic and Antitoxic Bolus	(177)
Bolus of Calculus Bovis for Purging the Heart–Fire	(177)
Bolus of Citri Grandis	(178)
Bolus of Rhei and Eupolyphaga seu Steleophaga	(179)
Bolus of Six Drugs Including Rehmannia	(181)
Bolus of Ten Powerful Tonics	(184)
Cow–bezoar Bolus for Clearing Away Heat of the Upper Part of the Body	(185)
Decoction for Clearing Away Pestilent Factors and Detoxification	(186)
Decoction for Clearing Heat in Ying System	(188)
Decoction for Strngthening Middle Jiao and Benefiting Vital Energy	(189)
Decoction of Arctii for Soothing Muscles	(191)
Decoction of Coptidis for Detoxification	(193)
Decoction of Cinnamomi Adding Cinnamomi	(194)
Decoction for General Antiphlogistic	(196)
Decoction for Purging Liver–fire and Eliminating Dampness	(197)
Golden Lock Bolus for Keep Kidney Essence	(199)
Zaizao Powder	(200)
Powder for Antiphlogosis	(202)

Pill of Six Miraculous Drugs	(204)
Decoction of Phragmitis	(206)
Powder of Lonicerae and Forsythiae	(207)
Powder of Ledebouriellae for Dispersing the Superficies	(209)
White Tiger Decoction	(211)
Decoction of Gypsum Fibrosum and Three Yellows	(212)
Decoction of Ginseng for Nourishing Qi and Ying	(213)
Ease Powder	(215)
Decoction of Aneglicae Pubescentis and Taxilli	(217)
Decoction for Pus Drainage and Relieving Pain	(219)
Xiaojin Pellet	(220)
Decoction for Warming Yang	(221)
Decoction of Persicae for Purgation	(223)
Major Decoction for Purging Down Digestive Qi	(224)
Major Decoction of Bupleurum	(226)
Pill of Stephaniae Tetrandrae, Zanthoxyli, Lepidii seu Descurainiae and Rhei	(227)
Powder of Bupleuri for Dispersing the Depressed Liver-Qi	(228)
Decoction of Gentianae for Purging Liver-Fire	(229)
Pulse-Activating Powder	(230)
Decoction for Rashes Subsidence	(231)
Decoction of Restoration	(233)
Decoction for Severe Phlegm-Heat Syndrome in the Chest	(234)
Decoction for Soothing the Intestine	(234)
Decoction of Angelicae Sinensis for Analgesic	(236)
Decoction of Angelicae Sinensis for Warming Cold Limbs	(237)
Bolus for Severe Endogenous Wind-Syndrome	(238)
Bolus of Arisaematis	(240)

Part One Nasal Diseases

Chapter One
Acute Rhinitis

Acute rhinitis is a very common disease. It is an acute infective inflammation of the nasal mucosa. It's clinical features are a feeling of burning heat in the nose, nasal obstruction, sneezing, rhinorrhea, headache, fever, etc.. It is called "*Shāng fēng bí sè*" (stuffy nose due to the attack by exogenous wind) in traditional Chinese medicine.

ETIOLOGY AND PATHOGENESIS

Wind, the causative factor of hundred diseases, often brings cold and heat to invade the lung system, attack the orifice of the nose, causing dysfunctions of the lung in clarifying and descending abilities, as well as nasal obstruction.

MAIN SYMPTOMS AND SIGNS

1. Nasal obstruction, obstructive nasal sound.
2. Watery nasal discharge, sneeze, constitutional discomfort.
3. About 7 to 10 days' duration.
4. Congestion and swelling in mucosa of the nasal cavity, watery and tenacious secretion in the nose.

MAIN POINTS OF DIAGNOSIS

1. The disease begins from one to three days after the attack of exogenous wind-cold. it gets cured within seven to fourteen days.
2. The patient has aversion to wind, fever, burning sensation in the nose, nasal obstruction, rhinocnesmus, sneezing an rhinorrhea. The nasal discharge is at first like clear water and then becomes sticky pus, or yellow pus in severe cases. Hyposmia may occur. Rhinolalia causa is present in speaking.
3. The mycric mucosa shows diffuse swelling and becomes scarlet win congestion. There is either lucid or pus-like sticky discharge in the nasal meatus.
4. There are accompanying symptoms such as cough with sputum, sore and itching throat, or tinnitus and hypoacusis.

DIFFERENTIATION AND TREATMENT OF COMMON SYNDROMES

1. Internal Treatment

1) **the type of he attack by exopathic wind-cold**

Main Symptoms and Signs: Stuffy nose and sneezing occur. The nasal discharge is thin and lucid, and edema of the nasal mucosa is present, accompanied by aversion to col, low fever, cough with white sputum as well as sore limbs. The tongue is light red, with thin and white fur and the pulse is floating and tight.

Therapeutic Principles: Dispelling pathogenic wind and col and removing obstruction from the upper orifices.

Recipe: *Sinyin san*

Flos Magnoliae	9 g
Rhizoma et Radix Ligustici	9 g
Rhizoma Cimicifugae	9 g
Rhizoma Ligustici Chuanxiong	9 g
Caulis Akebiae	9 g
Radix Ledebouriellae	9 g
Rhizoma seu Radix Notopterygii	9 g

Radix Angelicae Dahuricae	18 g
Radix Glycyrrhizae	6 g
Herba Asari	3 g

All the above drugs are to be decocted in water for oral administration.

Recipe 2: *Xing su san*

Semen Armeniacae Amarum	9 g
Radix Peucedani	9 g
Folium Perillae	12 g
Radix Platycodi	12 g
Exocarpium Citri Grandis	9 g
Rhizoma Pinelliae	9 g
Poria	12 g
Radix Glycyrrhizae	6 g
Fructus Aurantii	9 g
Rhizoma Zingiberis Recens	3 slices
Fructus Ziziphi Jujubae	6 pieces

All the above drugs are to be decocted in water for oral administration.

Modification: In case of severe cold, **Radix Ledebouriellae** 12 g and **Radix Puerariae** 30 g are added; for severe nasal obstruction, add **Radix Angelicae Dahuricae** 12 g and **Flos Magnoliae** 9 g.

Chinese Patent Medicine

Fufang daqingye heji. Take 10 ml each time, 3 times a day.

2) the type of the attack by exopathic wind-heat

Main Symptoms and Signs: The nose is obstructed with yellow and thick nasal discharge. There is a feeling of burning heat in the nose. The nasal mucosa is congested. There are throat, cough with yellow sputum and thirst. The tongue is red, with thin and yellow fur and the pulse is floating and rapid.

Therapeutic Principles: Disperse pathogenic wind and heat and remove obstruction from the upper orifices.

Recipe: *Decoction of mulberry leaf and chrysanthemum* and *Xanthium powder*

Frucus Xanthii	9 g
Flos Magnoliae	9 g
Flos Chrysanthemi	15 g

Rhizoma Phragmitis	15 g
Radix Angelicae Dahuricae	15 g
Fructus Forsythiae	15 g
Radix Glycyrrhizae	6 g

All the above drugs are to be decocted in water for oral administration.

Modification: For those who cough with profuse sputum, add 9 grams of *Rhizoma Pinelliae* and *Bulbus Fritillariae Cirrhosae* each, 15 grams of *Radix Asteris* and *Flos Farfarae* each. For those with sore throat, add 15 grams of *Radix Scutellariae* and 30 grams of *Flos Lonicerae*, 30 grams of *Herba Violae* and 12 grams o *Fructus Arctii*.

Chinese Patent Medicine

Xi ling jiedu pian. Take 6 tablets each time, 3 times a day. Lingyang ganmao pian. Take 6 tablets each time, 4 times a day. Ganmao chonji. Take 1 package each time. 3 times a day, and drink after it is stirred in boiled water.

2. External Treatment

1) Apply Congbai di bi ye, 3 times a day.
2. Drop the nose with Di bi ling, 3 times a day.

Acupuncture and Moxibustion

The acupoints are Yìntáng(EX − HN3), Tàiyáng(EX − HN5), Hégǔ(LI4), Fēngchí(GB20), Qūchí(LI11) and Zúsānlǐ(ST36). The acupoints are punctured with strong stimulation and with the needles retained for 10 to 15 minutes. The ignited moxa−stick is supposed to heat Yíngxiāng(LI20) and Shàngxīng(DU23) till local skin becomes warm.

Chapter Two
Chronic Rhinitis

Chronic rhinitis is a chronic inflammatory change o the nasal mucosa, mainly due to the protraction of acute rhinitis. Its main symptom is nasal obstruction. This disease is called "Bí zhì" (nasal obstruction) in traditional Chinese medicine.

ETIOLOGY AND PATHOGENESIS

It is related to *qi* deficiency of the lung and spleen which fails o protect the body from being attacked by pathogenic factors, and which leaves the evils and toxins to linger in the body, resulting in accumulation of the evils in meridians and collaterals, stagnation of *qi* and *blood* as well as nasal obstruction.

MAIN SYMPTOMS AND SIGNS

1. Intermittent, alternative or continuous nasal obstruction.
2. Swelling or hypertrophy of nasal mucosa, which is as big as mulberry fruit and in dark-red color, especially in inferior nasal concha.

MAIN POINTS OF DIAGNOSIS

1. The nasal obstruction is either alternate, intermittent or continuous.
2. The nasal mucosa swells or becomes thick, especially that of the inferior nasal concha.
3. Hyposmia is fluctuating.
4. There is pain and itching in the throat and tinnitus or hypoacusis may occur.

DIFFERENTIATION AND TREATMENT OF COMMON SYNDROMES

1. Internal Treatment

the type of qi – deficiency of both the lung and the spleen

Main Symptoms and Signs: The nasal obstruction is relieved in the morning and aggravated at night and becomes severer if exposed to cold. When the patient lies in lateral recumbent position, it is less severe in the upper part than in the lower one, or becomes alternate. The inferior nasal concha swells and has slight congestion. The conchae may contract if vasoconstrictor is used. There may be accompanying cough with thin sputum, short breath and asthenia. The tongue is light red, its fur white and the pulse moderate.

Therapeutic Principles: Strengthen the spleen, warm the lung, remove cold and clear away he obstruction from the upper orifices.

Recipe: *Pill for warming the lung to stop running nose* with additional ingredients

Radix Ginseng	6 – 9 g
Herba Schizonepetae	9 g
Fructus Chebulae	9 g
Radix Platycodi	9 g
Otolith Pseudosciaenae	15 g
Radix Angelicae Dahuricae	15 g
Herba Asari	3 g
Radix Glycyrrhizae	6 g
Radix Astragali seu Hedysari	24 g

All the above drugs are to be decocted in water for oral administration.

Modification: For severe spleen qi deficiency, add *Radix Astragali seu Hedysari* 18 g, *Rhizoma Atractylodis Macrocephalae* 15 g. For cough and profuse sputum, add *Bulbus Fritillariae Cirrhosae* 9 g and *Rhizoma Cynanchi Stauntonii* 12 g.

Chinese Patent Medicine

Qianbai biyang pian. Take 4 tablets each time orally, 3 times a day. Reduce the dosage with the symptoms relieved.

Huo dan wan: Take 6 grams each time, 3 times a day.

Biyan pian: Take 4 tablets each time, 3 times a day.

the type of stagnation of qi and blood stasis

Main Symptoms and Signs: The patient has continuous nasal obstruction and hyposmia. The inferior nasal concha is hypertrophic and dark red or like moruloid and insensitive to vasoconstrictor. There are accompanying symptoms such as is red or has petechiae on it. The pulse is taut and uneven.

Therapeutic Principles: Promote *blood* circulation to remove blood stasis and resolving masses to clear away obstruction from the upper orifices.

Recipe: *Peach kernel and safflower decoction of four ingredients*, combined with *Xanthium Powder*

Semen Persicae	9 g
Flos Carthami	9 g
Radix Rehmanniae	9 g
Frucus Xanthii	9 g
Herba Menthae	9 g
Flos Magnoliae	9 g
Radix Angelicae Sinensis	15 g
Radix Paeoniae Rubra	15 g
Rhizoma Ligustici Chuanxiong	12 g
Radix Angelicae Dahuricae	18 g

All the above drugs are to be decocted in water for oral administration.

Modification: For those with severe nasal obstruction, add 9 grams of *Spina Gleditsiae* and *Squama Manitis* each. For those with headache, add 9 grams of **Rhizoma et Radix Ligustici** and **Fructus Viticis** each. For those who have severe *blood* stasis, add 9 grams of **Rhizoma Sparganii** and **Rhizoma Zedoariae** each. For those who have shortness of breath and asthenia, add 15 g of **Radix Codonopsis Pilosulae**, 9 grams of **Rhizoma Atractylodis Macrocephalae** and 9 grams of **Fructus Amomi**.

yin deficiency o the lung and kidney

Main Symptoms and Signs: Dryness and a sensation of obstruction in the nose, hyposmia, blood threads in the nasal discharge, fetor narium, dry throat, dry cough with little sputum, feverish sensation in the palms and soles. Red tongue with little coating, thready and rapid pulse.

Therapeutic Principles: Nourish the lung and replenish the kidney.

Recipe:

Radix Rehmanniae	15 g
Radix Scrophulariae	12 g
Radix Ophiopogonis	12 g
Bulbus Fritillariae	9 g
Radix Platycodi	9 g
Cortex Moutan	9 g
Herba Menthae	6 g
Radix Glycyrrhizae	6 g

Chinese Patent Medicine

Lily lung-strengthening pill. Take 8 pills each time orally, 3 times a day.

accumulated heat in the lung meridian

Main Symptoms and Signs: Profuse yellow turbid nasal discharge, long duration of nasal obstruction, hyposmia, dizziness, distention in the head, hypomnesia. Red tongue with yellow coating, wiry and thready pulse.

Therapeutic Principles: Clear away heat, promote the dispersing function of the lung and open the orifice.

Recipe:

Frucus Xanthii	9 g
Flos Magnoliae	9 g
Rhizoma Anemarrhenae	9 g
Rhizoma Cimicifugae	9 g
Herba Menthae	6 g
Fructus Gardeniae	12 g
Gypsum Fibrosum	30 g
Radix Angelicae Dahuricae	15 g

Chinese Patent Medicine

Agasache and Pig's bile tablets. Take 5 tablets each time orally, 3 times a day.

2. External Treatment

1) Use *Effectual nose dip* for nasal drip. This should be done three times a

day.

2) Blow *Powder of eardust of yellow coaker* into nasal cavity. its ingredients are as follows:

Otolith Pseudosciaenae	9 g
Borneolum Syntheticum	0.9 g
Flos Magnoliae	6 g
Herba Asari	3 g

All the above drugs are to be decocted in water for oral administration.

3) Massage he nasal part. Knead with two thumbs to and fro along the back of the nose until a sensation of enough heat is produced. Do this twice a day.

4) **simpel and convenient recipe**

Add a little borneol into some *sesame oil* and use the mixture for nasal dip three times daily. It is suitable o the patients with *yin* deficiency o both lung and kidney.

Acupuncture and Moxibustion

1. **Body Acupuncture**

Main Points: **Yíngxiāng(LI20), Yìntáng(EX－HN3), Lièquē(LU7), Hégǔ(LI4), Dàzhuī(DU14)**, and **Fēngmén(BL12)**.

Complementary Points: Add **Tàiyáng(EX－HN5)** for headache.

Manipulation: Puncture the points with filiform needles and retain them for 20 minutes. The seed－embedding method or subcutaneous needle is also applicable.

3) Injection Therapy: 0.5 ml of *Danggui zhushe ye* is supposed to inject into **Yíngxiāng(LI20)**, once every other day, five injections as one course.

4) Moxibustion: The points are **Shuǐgōu(DB), Yíngxiāng(LI20), Fēngfǔ(DU16), Fèishū(BL13)** in case of *qi* deficiency; **Píshū(BL20)** (for spleen deficiency) and **Zúsānlǐ(ST36)**. Moxibustion is supposed to heat the acupoints till local skin feels warm.

MASSAGE

Press and knead **Bǎihuì(DU20), Shàngxīng(DU23), Yìntáng(EX－HN3)**

Chronic Rhinitis

Yíngxiāng(LI20) 30 times respectively. Chafe along the sides o nose 30 times. Rub the hands and wash the face for 50 times. Grasp and knead **Hégǔ**(LI4) 30 times respectively, and pinch **Shàoshāng**(LU11) 20 times.

Medicated Diet

1. Have one duck rid of its feathers and internal organs. Put the duck with 15 g of *Chinses caterpillar fungus* in its belly, in a plate with just the right amount of water. Steam it over the boiling water until the duck is done. Take the duck and soup.

2. Cook gruel with 60 g of *polished round - grained rice*, 20 g of *Semen Phaseoli Radiati* and 15 g of *lily bulb*. Add some *crystal sugar* just as the gruel is half done. Take one dose a day for 10 days totally.

Qigong

1. Wash the face

Two hands are rubbed hot, then rub the lateral sides of the nose upwards with middle fingers; while reaching the forehead, then rub two cheeks downwards with two hands. It can be repeated 9 times. This can promote the smooth flow of *qi* and *blood* on the face and prevent common cold.

2. Rub the nose

The index fingers are piled up on the middle fingers. The middle fingers are pressed on the lateral sides of the nose to rub the nose upwards and downwards. Then the thumb knuckles are placed on **Yíngxiāng**(LI20) to knead them 20 times. The method can prevent common cold and dredge the obstructed nasal cavity.

Chapter Three
Allergic Rhinitis

Allergic rhinitis is an allergic disease caused by the sensitinogen acting on the mucous membranes of the nasal cavity, also called perennial allergic rhinitis. Clinically it has the following features: itching in the nose, sneeze, watery nasal discharge, nasal obstruction coming and going suddenly. It is called "Bí qíu", a reference to allergic rhinitis.

ETIOLOGY AND PATHOGENESIS

It is related to invasion of allergic evils which cause dysfunction o the lung in descending and dispersing abilities, and dysfunction of the kidney in governing and accepting abilities, resulting in internal production of turbid dampness, accumulation of body fluid, lingering nasal discharge.

MAIN SYMPTOMS AND SIGNS

1. Tickling sensation in the nose, accompanied by tickling sensation in the eyes and throat, nasal obstruction.
2. Frequent sneeze, often over ten continuous sneezes during a rather short period of time.
3. Nasal discharge, profuse watery secretion.
4. Paroxysmal attack of above-mentioned symptoms, with rapid onset and disappearance, reoccurrence and intractability.
5. Pale or grayish blue color in nasal mucosa with obvious swelling, moisture and softness to the touch, mulberry fruit-like affection in inferior nasal concha in lingering cases, or polypoid affection in middle nasal concha, profuse watery secretion in meatus nasi medius or meatus nasi communis.
6. Slight red tongue, thin and white tongue coating, thready and feeble

Allergic Rhinitis

pulse.

7. Pale facial complexion, lassitude, shortness o breath, reluctance of speaking, or poor appetite, loose stool, aversion to cold, cold sensation in limbs, soreness in low back, frequent nocturnal urination.

MAIN POINTS OF DIAGNOSIS

1. Itching in the nasal cavity occurs suddenly, accompanied with itching in the eyes and pharynx.

2. The patient has one sneeze after another, sometimes dozens of them in succession.

3. There is watery nasal discharge with foams. In the period of acute reaction, plenty of nasal discharge comes out continuously.

4. At the beginning the nasal obstruction is transient. Then it becomes continuous, or accompanied with hyposmia.

5. The mucous membrane in the nasal cavity (chiefly in the middle and inferior conchae) shows swelling, pale or grayish blue in color, and moist and pliable. In the course of time, moruloid change in the inferior concha or a polypoid change in the middle concha will occur, with a lot of watery secretion in the nasal meatus.

DIFFERENTIATION AND TREATMENT OF COMMON SYNDROMES

1. Internal Treatment

1) deficiency of spleen qi

Main Symptoms and Signs: The patient has paroxysmal itching, sore and swelling in the nose, sneezes with much watery nasal discharge, intermittent nasal obstruction and pale nasal mucosa with local swelling, accompanied with tiredness or asthenia, deficiency in breath and no desire for talking, poor appetite, loose stool, aversion to cold and cool limbs, sore in the loins and frequent urination at night. The tongue is light red, with thin and white fur and the pulse is thready.

Therapeutic Principles: Strengthen the spleen, replenish qi and disperse pathogenic cold to remove obstruction from the upper orifices.

Recipe: *Decoction for reinforcing middle — jiao and replenishing qi compounded with Xanthium powder*

Radix Astragali seu Hedysari	18 g
Radix Ginseng	9 g
Radix Angelicae Sinensis	9 g
Frucus Xanthii	9 g
Flos Magnoliae	9 g
Herba Menthae	9 g
Rhizoma Cimicifugae	9 g
Pericarpium Citri Reticulatae	9 g
Rhizoma Atractylodis Macrocephalae	9 g
Radix Glycyrrhizae Praeparata	9 g
Radix Bupleuri	9 g
Radix Angelicae Dahuricae	15 g

All the above drugs are to be decocted in water for oral administration.

Modification: For those with apparent manifestations of deficiency of the lung qi, increase the dosage of *Radix Astragali seu Hedysari* to 30 grams and add 9 grams of *Radix Ledebouriellae* to the recipe. For those with accompanying abdominal distention and loose stool, add 15 grams of *Semen Dolichoris Album* and 18 grams of *Semen Coicis*. For those with soreness in the loins and frequent urination a night, add 6 grams of *Rhizoma Curculiginis*, 9 grams of *Radix Aconiti Praeparata* or use additionally *Golden chamber bolus for tonifying kidney — qi*. For those who have hypertrophic inferior nasal concha, add 15 grams of *Radix Paeoniae Rubra*, 9 grams of *Rhizoma Ligustici Chuanxiong* and 9 grams of *Fructus Liquidambaris*. For those who have plenty of watery nasal discharge, add 9 grams of *Fructus Schisandrae*, 9 grams of *Fructus Mume* and 3 grams of *Herba Asari*.

2) **attack by pathogenic wind**

Main Symptoms and Signs: Paroxysmal itching, sore and distending sensation in the nose, sneezes with much watery nasal discharge, accompanied by cough, a little sputum, sore throat and headache. Red tongue with thin and white coating, floating pulse.

Therapeutic Principles: Expel wind and open the upper orifice.

Recipe:

Folium Mori	9 g
Radix Platycodi	6 g
Frucus Xanthii	9 g
Flos Magnoliae	9 g
Radix Angelicae Dahuricae	15 g
Radix Ledebouriellae	9 g
Radix Glycyrrhizae	3 g

All the above drugs are to be decocted in water for oral administration.

Chinese Patent Medicine

Rhinitis tablet. Take 4 tablets each time, 3 times a day.

3) **deficiency of lung** *qi*

Main Symptoms and Signs: Intermittent nasal obstruction, pale nasal mucosa with local swelling, accompanied by shortness of breath, no desire for talking, poor appetite, tiredness, aversion to cold and cold limbs. Pale tongue with thin and white coating, thready pulse.

Therapeutic Principles: Strengthen the lung and replenish *qi* and open the upper orifice.

Recipe:

Radix Astragali seu Hedysari	30 g
Radix Rehmanniae	12 g
Radix Ophiopogonis	15 g
Bulbus Fritillariae	9 g
Herba Menthae	6 g
Rhizoma Curculiginis	9 g
Radix Glycyrrhizae Praeparata	6 g

Chinese Patent Medicine

1) *Jade wind - barrier infusion*. Take one packet each time after being infused in boiling water, twice a day.

2) *Bi yan pian*. Take 4 tablets each time, 3 times daily.

3) *Huo dan wan*. Take 6 g each time, 3 times a day.

4) *Jingui shenqi wan*. Take one pill each time, 3 times a day.

5) *Yun zhi gan tai zhongji*. Take one package with boiled water each tim, 3 times a day.

2. External Treatment

1) Blow *Biyun powder* into the nose. Its ingredients are as follows:

Herba Centipedae	30 g
Rhizoma Ligustici Chuanxiong	30 g
Flos Magnoliae	6 g
Herba Asari	6 g
Indigo Naturalis	3 g

Grind the above drugs together into fine powder and blow it into the nose three times a day.

2) Insert into the nose *Ointment tablet of eardust of yellow croaker*. The ingredients are as follows:

Recipe:

Otolith Pseudosciaenae	9 g
Borneolum Syntheticum	0.9 g
Flos Magnoliae	6 g
Herba Asari	3 g

Grind the above drugs together into fine powder and add quantum sufficit of Vaseline to make ointment tablets from it. Insert one ointment tablet in the nose each day.

Acupuncture and Moxibustion

1. body acupuncture

Main Points: **Lièquē**(LU7), **Hégǔ**(LI4), **Yíngxiāng**(LI20), and **Yìntáng**(EX-HN3).

Complemenatary Points: Add **Tàiyáng**(EX-HN5) for headache.

Manipulation: Apply filiform needles with sedation and retain the needles for 15 minutes, and manipulate them once or twice in interval.

Auricular Acupuncture

Prescribed Points: inner nose, forehead, lung, adrenal gland, and asthma.

Allergic Rhinitis

Manipulation: 2 – 3 points are selected each time. The filiform needles are applied with strong stimulation and retained for 30 minutes. The seed – embedding method or subcutaneous needle is also applicable.

MASSAGE

Press and knead **Fēngchí**(GB20), **Fēngmén**(BL12), **Tàiyáng**(EX – HN5) and **Yìntáng**(EX – HN3) 30 times respectively. Push the forehead divergently for 30 times. Press and knead **Yíngxiāng**(LI20) 50 times. Scrub along the sides of the nose 30 times. Pat the upper part of the back 30 times. Knead **Dǎnzhōng**(RN17) 30 times. Scrub **Dàzhuī**(DU14) 30 times and press and knead **Hégǔ**(LI4) 30 times.

Medicated Diet

Wash 50 g of *polished round – grained rice* and put it in a cooking pot. Add right amount of water and heat it over a strong fire until it boils. Then boil it to a low fire for 40 minutes. Put in 50 g of *lily bulbs* and go on cooling until it is done. Add *crystal sugar* before eating. Take the gruel once in the morning and in the evening respectively.

Qigong

Assume the sitting or standing posture. Get rid of nasal discharge. Relax and tranquilize the body naturally and breathe evenly. Rub the dorsa of both thumbs against each other until they are warm. Then slightly rub the two sides of the nose. Rub for 5 times in inhalation and 5 times in exhalation. Do 6 breaths altogether.

Press the tip of the middle finger of the right hand on the apex of the nose. Move leftward in circular motion for 5 times in inhalation and rightward for 5 times in exhalation. Do 6 times altogether.

Chapter Four
Rhinitis Sicca

Rhinitis sicca refers to the condition caused by dryness and lack of fluid in the nasal mucosa. In traditional Chinese medicine, it is called "Bí zào" (nasal dryness).

ETIOLOGY AND PATHOGENESIS

It is related to invasion of pathogenic wind, heat, summer heat and dryness which ascend and attack the nose, causing lack of nourishment in the nasal mucosa.

MAIN SYMPTOMS AND SIGNS

1. Dryness in nasal cavity, decreased secretion, intermittent dry pain, tickling sensation. The patient often scratches and kneads the nose for alleviating symptoms and sometimes it would cause slight nasal bleeding.

2. Dryness and congestion in nasal mucosa, erosion on mucous epithelium of the anteroinferior nasal septum, even ulceration, no atrophy in nasal mucosa and various nasal concha.

3. Accompanied by thirst, dry throat, cough with a little sputum, poor appetite, abdominal distention, pale complexion, or warm sensation in five centers, dream-disturbed sleep, red tongue, thin and white tongue coating, superficial pulse.

DIFFERENTIATION AND TREATMENT OF COMMON SYNDROMES

1. Internal Treatment

Therapeutic Principles: Replenish *yin* and nourish *blood*; clean the lung and moisten dryness.

Recipe: *Yang yin qing fei tang*

Radix Rehmanniae	15 g
Radix Ophiopogonis	18 g
Radix Paeoniae Alba	12 g
Cortex Moutan Radicis	12 g
Bulbus Fritillariae Cirrhosae	9 g
Radix Scrophulariae	15 g
Herba Menthae	9 g
Radix Glycyrrhizae	6 g

All the above drugs are to be decocted in water for oral administration.

Modification: In case of dry nose with splitting pain, add *Rhizoma Phragmitis* 15 g and *Radix Adenophora Tetraphylla* 18 g. For nasal bleeding, add *Nodus Nelumbinis Rhizomatis* 15 g and *Rhizoma Imperatae* 15 g. For warm sensation in five centers, add *Radix Asparagi* 12 g and *Fructus Mori* 24 g. In case of poor appetite and loose stools, add *Radix Ginseng* 6 g and *Rhizoma Atractylodis Macrocephalae* 15 g, and *Poria* 12 g.

2. External Treatment

1) Drop nose with sesame oil added by a little *Borneolum Syntheticum*, 4 times a day.

2) Drop nose with *Fufang bohe you*, 3 times a day.

3) Blow *Yu nao shi san* into the nose, twice to 3 times a day.

Acupuncture and Moxibustion

Body Acupuncture: Yíngxiāng (LI20), Kǒuhéliáo (LI19), and Sùliáo (DU25), etc., can be punctured perpendicularly and obliquely with the needles retained for

10 to 15 minutes.

Auricular Acupuncture: It is advisable to embed *Semen Vaccariae* on the points internal nose, external nose, lung, endocrine and subcortex, etc., on both auricles alternatively every other day.

3) **Moxibustion:** It is applicable to heat **Bǎihuì(DU20)** and **Zúsānlǐ(ST36)** with moxa-stick till local skin feels warm and becomes red in color, once every other day.

Chapter Five
Atrophic Rhinitis

Atrophic rhinitis is a chronic atrophic change of the nasal mucosa, periost and nasal conchae. Its clinical features are dryness in the nose, nasal widened nasal cavity with crusts on it, coryza foetida and hyposmia. This disease occurs mostly in young females. In traditional Chinese medicine it is called "Bí gǎo" (a reference to atrophic rhinitis).

ETIOLOGY AND PATHOGENESIS

The lung is considered as a tender organ and likes moisture and dislikes dryness. If attacked by pathogenic dryness, it would present dry nose, or it is related to spleen *qi* deficiency which leads to disability of fluid transportation and is unable to moisten the nasal cavity; or related to *yin* deficiency in the kidney which fails to distribute body fluid upwards for nourishing the nose, all of which would cause *yin* deficiency and consumption of body fluid.

MAIN SYMPTOMS AND SIGNS

1. Dry nose, burning pain, nasal obstruction.
2. Stinking odor in the nose, crustae, yellowish purulent and turbid nasal discharge, or bloody nasal discharge.
3. Hyposmia or anosmia.
4. Enlargement of nasal cavity, atrophy of nasal mucosa and concha, yellowish and purulent crustae; dry and thin mucosa with erosion, dark and lustrousless color or bleeding spots after decrustation.

MAIN POINTS OF DIAGNOSIS

1. There is dryness in the nose and a feeling of obstruction in the nasal cavity. The nasal discharge is yellow – green and full of crusts, or coryza foetida may occur in severe cases.

2. Hyposmia may occur. In severe cases, anosmia may be present.

3. The nasal cavity is widened and the nasal mucosa is dry and covered with yellow – green crusts of nasal discharge. After the crusts are removed, superficial erosion on the membrane can be seen. The nasal conchae become atrophic and even indiscernible in severe cases.

4. In severe cases the nose becomes flat with its wings bent.

5. There is dryness in the nasopharynx or in the pharynx. An examination shows that the pharyngeal mucosa is dry or atrophic.

DIFFERENTIATION AND TREATMENT OF COMMON SYNDROMES

1. Internal Treatment

1) the type of dryness of the lung due to yin – deficiency

Main Symptoms and Signs: There are such symptoms as dryness, redness, a sensation of obstruction in the nose, dryness of the nasal mucosa covered with crusts of nasal discharge, hyposmia, accompanied by dry throat and cough due to itching in the pharynx, red and uncoated tongue and thready and rapid pulse.

Therapeutic Principles: Nourish yin to moisten the lung.

Recipe: *Decoction for nourishing yin and clearing away lung – heat*

Radix Rehmanniae	15 g
Radix Ophiopogonis	15 g
Radix Paeoniae Alba	15 g
Cortex Moutan Radicis	
Bulbus Fritillariae Cirrhosae	9 g
Radix Scrophulariae	9 g
Herba Menthae	9 g
Radix Glycyrrhizae	6 g

All the above drugs are to be decocted in water for oral administration.

2) the type of deficiency and weakness of both the lung and the kidney

Main Symptoms and Signs: There are such symptoms as dryness in the nasopharynx and a feeling of stuffiness in the nose, anosmia, fetor narium, widened nasal cavity with erosion on the mucous membrane covered with yellow – green crusts, blood threads in the nasal discharge. In severe cases, the nose bridge becomes low and flat. The accompanying symptoms are mental fatigue, asthenia, feverish sensation in the palms and soles, dry cough with little sputum, tinnitus and dreaminess, red tongue with little fur and thready and rapid pulse.

Therapeutic Principles: Reinforce and replenish the lung and kidney.

Recipe: *Lily decoction for strengthening the lung*

Radix Rehmanniae	15 g
Radix Ophiopogonis	15 g
Radix Paeoniae Alba	15 g
Radix Angelicae Sinensis	15 g
Radix Scrophulariae	15 g
Radix Rehmanniae Praeparata	18 g
Bulbus Lillii	18 g
Bulbus Fritillariae Cirrhosae	9 g
Radix Platycodi	9 g
Radix Glycyrrhizae Praeparata	6 g

All the above drugs are to be decocted in water for oral administration.

Modification: For those with dryness and sore in the nasopharynx, add 15 grams of **Herba Dendrobii**, **Radix Adenophorae**, and **Rhizoma Polygonati Odorati**. For those with *blood* in he nasal discharge, add 9 grams of **Radix Scutellariae**, 30 grams of **Herba Agrimoniae** and 30 grams of **Rhizoma Imperatae**. For those with severe atrophy of the nasal conchae, add 30 grams of **Radix Salviae Miltiorrhizae** and 15 grams of **Herba Cistanchis**.

Chinese Patent Medicine

1) *Zhi bai dihuang wan*. Take one pill each time, 3 times a day.
2) *Liu wei dihuang wan*: Take one pill each time, 3 times a day.

3) **lung – *yin* deficiency**

Main Symptoms and Signs: Severe dryness in the nose, nasal obstruction with tickling sensation, burning pain, hyposmia, atrophy of muscular membrane in the nose, turbid nasal discharge in yellow and purulent color, crustae, cough, tickling sensation in the throat, dry mouth, red tongue, scanty tongue coating, thready and rapid pulse.

Therapeutic Principles: Nourish yin and moisten dryness for assisting the lung in dispersing ability and expelling evils.

Recipe: *Qing zao jiu fei tang*

Folium Mori	12 g
Gypsum Fibrosum	24 g
Colla Corii Asini	9 g
Radix Ophiopogonis	15 g
Semen Sesami Indici	9 g
Radix Codonopsis Pilosulae	15 g
Radix Glycyrrhizae	6 g
Semen Armeniacae Amarum	9 g
Folium Eriobotryae	12 g

All the above drugs are to be decocted in water for oral administration.

Modification: For severe dry nose and mouth, add *Radix Adenophora Tetraphylla* 15 g and *Herba Dendrobii* 12 g. In case of epistaxis, add *Cacumen Biotae* 15 g and *Cortex Moutan Radicis* 12 g.

Chinese Patent Medicine

Yang yin qing fei wan. Take one pill each time, 3 times a day.

4) **spleen qi deficiency**

Main Symptoms and Signs: Dryness in the nose, stinking nasal discharge, yellow and purulent crustae, anosmia, enlargement and severe atrophy of nasal cavity, accompanied by serious headache, poor appetite, abdominal distention, lassitude, pale tongue, thin and white tongue coating, slow and feeble pulse.

Therapeutic Principles: Nourish the middle jiao and benefit *qi*; tonify *yin* and moisten dryness.

Recipe:

Radix Astragali seu Hedysari	18 g
Radix Glycyrrhizae	6 g

Radix Codonopsis Pilosulae	15 g
Radix Angelicae Sinensis	12 g
Pericarpium Citri Reticulatae	12 g
Rhizoma Cimicifugae	6 g
Radix Bupleuri	12 g
Radix Angelicae Dahuricae	15 g
Radix Rehmanniae Praeparata	12 g
Radix Paeoniae Alba	15 g
Rhizoma Ligustici Chuanxiong	9 g

All the above drugs are to be decocted in water for oral administration.

Modification: For stinking odor in the nose, add *Cortex Phellodendri* 9 g and *Herba Agastachis* 12 g. For anosmia, add *Herba Menthae* 9 g and *Flos Magnoliae* 9 g.

Chinese Patent Medicine

Renshen jian pi wan. Take one pill each time, 3 times a day.

2. External Treatment

1) Use *Nose drops of desertliving cistache*. Its ingredients are as follows:

Herba Cistanchis	300 g
Folium Epimedii	300 g
Radix Angelicae Sinensis	300 g
Ramulus Cinnamomi	300 g
Radix Astragali seu Hedysari	300 g

All the above drugs are decocted in water twice and then the decoction is concentrated into an extract which is to be mixed with 500 ml of *parafin oil*. Use the mixture for nasal drip, three times a day.

2) Use *Nose drops of sesame oil*. Add a little *borneol* into some *sesame oil* and use the mixture for nasal drip twice a day.

3) Steam 9 g of *Flos Chrysanthemi Alba* and 6 g of *Mel* together for two hours, and remove *Flos Chrysanthemi* and drop the nose with medicated honey,

3 times a day.

4) Soak 9 g of *Rhizoma Coptidis* into 90 g of *sesame oil* for seven days, and then drop nose with this medicated oil, 3 times daily.

Chapter Six
Acute Nasosinusitis

*A*cute nasosinusitis is an acute nonspecific inflammation of the mucous membrane of the frontal sinus, ethmoid sinus and maxillary sinus (sphenoiditis is seldom seen). Its clinical characteristics are fever, headache, nasal obstruction and purulent nasal discharge. It belongs to the category of "Bí yuān" (rhinorrhea with turbid discharge) in traditional Chinese medicine.

ETIOLOGY AND PATHOGENESIS

It is related to the pathogenic factors which invade and attack the human body and mix with the heat in the lung, spleen and gallbladder, ascending to the orifice of the nose, steaming and burning the muscular membrane of the nasal sinuses.

MAIN SYMPTOMS AND SIGNS

1. Decrease of smelling ability in the attack of nasal obstruction.
2. Profuse and purulent nasal discharge at the initial time yellow and white thick nasal discharge, and then yellow, turbid and tenacious nasal discharge with stinking odor and difficulty to blow of.
3. Splitting headache or distention and discomfort in the head. headache varies with the condition of sick sinuses, mostly appearing in the superficial skull in sinusitis of the anterior group of sinuses or in deep location in sinusitis of posterior group of sinuses.
4. There is painful sensation from percussion on the surface of projection of sinuses. There are obvious congestion and swelling in the nasal mucosa, especially severe redness and swelling in the middle nasal concha; there is a large volume of tenacious purulent secretion can be seen in meatus concha ethmoturbinalis majoris

and rhinal fissure after nasal discharge is blown out.

MAIN POINTS OF DIAGNOSIS

1. Mostly the patient has a history of upper respiratory tract infection or of being choked in water when swimming.

2. The patient has headache or pain in the area of nasal sinuses which may be distending, stabbing or jumping and may occur at a specific time (for instance in the case of maxillary sinusitis or frontal sinusitis, mild in the morning, severe at noon and gradually relieved again in the afternoon). Examination will find tenderness in the corresponding areas of the nasal sinuses.

3. The nasal obstruction is alternate or intermittent, and accompanied with hyposmia.

4. There is much sticky or yellow purulent nasal discharge.

5. The nasal mucosa swells, with purulent secretion flowing out from or accumulating in the nasal meatus to which the relevant sinuses open.

X-ray photograph shows that the corresponding nasal sinuses are of low degree of transparency and there is cloudiness or fluid level (take maxillary sinusitis for instance).

7. There are general symptoms such as aversion to cold, running fever and being uncomfortable all over.

DIFFERENTIATION AND TREATMENT OF COMMON SYNDROMES

1. Internal Treatment

1) the attack of wind-heat on the lung channel

Main Symptoms and Signs: The nose is obstructed, with the nasal discharge sticky in nature and white or yellow in color. The mucous membrane of the nasal cavity becomes red with swelling. Pus accumulates in the nasal meatus. The accompanying symptoms are fever, aversion to wind and headache. The tongue fur is thin and yellow and the pulse floating and rapid.

Therapeutic Principles: Disperse pathogenic wind, clear away pathogenic heat and ventilate the lung to remove obstruction from the upper orifices.

Recipe: *Xanthium powder* compounded with *Powder of lonicera and forsythia*

Frucus Xanthii	9 g
Flos Magnoliae	9 g
Herba Schizonepetae	9 g
Semen Sojae Praeparatum	9 g
Fructus Arctii	9 g
Folium Bambusae	9 g
Herba Menthae	9 g
Radix Angelicae Dahuricae	18 g
Flos Lonicerae	18 g
Rhizoma Phragmitis	18 g
Radix Glycyrrhizae	6 g
Radix Platycodi	6 g

All the above drugs are to be decocted in water for oral administration.

Recipe: *Qing kong gao*

Radix Scutellariae	15 g
Radix Ledebouriellae	15 g
Rhizoma seu Radix Notopterygii	9 g
Rhizoma Coptidis	12 g
Radix Bupleuri	15 g
Rhizoma Ligustici Chuanxiong	9 g
Radix Glycyrrhizae	6 g

All the above drugs are to be decocted in water for oral administration.

Modification: For cough and profuse sputum, add *Semen Armeniacae Amarum* 9 g, *Folium Eriobotryae* 12 g. For severe nasal obstruction, add *Radix Angelicae Dahuricae* 15 and *Flos Magnoliae* 9 g. For excessive yellow and turbid nasal discharge, add *Herba Houttuyniae* 15 g and *Spina Gleditsiae* 15 g. In cases with headache, the added drugs can be chosen in accordance with locations of headache. For vertex headache, add *Rhizoma et Radix Ligustici* 9 g. For frontal headache and pain in the superciliary ridge, add *Radix Angelicae Dahuricae* 15 g and *Fructus Viticis* 12 g. For occipital headache and neck pain, add *Radix Puerariae* 24 g. For temporal headache, add *Radix Bupleuri* 12 g and *Cortex Moutan Radicis* 12 g.

2) the intense heat in the gallbladder meridian

Main Symptoms and Signs: The nose is obstructed and the head aches terribly. The is yellow and turbid nasal discharge in the nose which gives a stinking odor. The mucous membrane of the nasal cavity swells and turns red. There is a lo of yellow pus-like discharge in the nasal meatus. The accompanying symptoms are fever, bitter taste in the mouth, dry throat, dysphoria and dizziness. The tongue is red, with yellow fur and the pulse taut and rapid.

Therapeutic Principles: Clear away pathogenic heat in the gallbladder meridian and eliminate turbid nasal discharge to remove obstruction from the upper orifices.

Recipe: *Decoction of gentiana for purging liver-fire*

Radix Gentianae	9 g
Radix Scutellariae	9 g
Radix Bupleuri	9 g
Radix Angelicae Sinensis	9 g
Rhizoma Alismatis	9 g
Fructus Gardeniae	15 g
Radix Rehmanniae	15 g
Semen Plantaginis (decocted after being wrapped in a piece of cloth)	15 g
Radix Glycyrrhizae	6 g
Caulis Akebiae	6 g

All the above drugs are to be decocted in water for oral administration.

3) dampness-heat in the spleen meridian

Main Symptoms and Signs: Nasal obstruction is continuous with much yellow turbid nasal discharge flowing out from the nose. The osphresis is obtuse. The nasal mucosa is distinctly red and swollen. There may be accompanying headache, fever, a sensation of heaviness in the head which seems to have been wrapped up, a feeling of distention in the stomach, loss of appetite and dark-red urine. The tongue is red, with yellow and greasy fur and the pulse is slippery and rapid.

Therapeutic Principles: Clear away heat and dampness and remove turbid nasal discharge and obstruction from the orifices.

Recipe: *Sweet dew detoxication pill*

Herba Artemisiae Scopriae	9 g
Radix Scutellariae	9 g
Rhizoma Acori Graminei	9 g
Rhizoma Ligustici Chuanxiong	
Rhizoma Belamcandae	9 g
Herba Menthae	9 g
Fructus Amomi Rotundus	9 g
Herba Agastachis seu Pogostemonis	9 g
Fructus Forsythiae	15 g
Caulis Akebiae	6 g

All the above drugs are to be decocted in water for oral administration.

Modification: For those with obvious headache, different herbs are to be added according to the location of the pain. For instance, those with parietal headache should use additionally 9 grams of *Rhizoma et Radix Ligustici*; those with ache in the supraorbital bone should add 18 grams of *Radix Angelicae Dahuricae*; those with occipital and nuchal headache should add 30 grams of *Radix Puerariae*; those with ache in the temple should add 9 grams of *Radix Bupleuri* and 9 grams of *Fructus Viticis*; those with ache in he facio – buccal region should add 9 grams of *Rhizoma Ligustici Chuanxiong* and 9 grams of *Radix Angelicae Dahuricae*; those with lot of pus – like nasal discharge should add 9 grams of *Herba Houttuyniae*, 9 grams of *Bulbus Fritillariae Thunbergii* and 9 grams of *Frucus Xanthii* and those with severe nasal obstruction should add 9 grams of *Cortex Moutan Radicis*, 9 grams of *Radix Paeoniae Rubra* and 3 grams of *Herba Asari*.

Recipe: Huangqin huashi tang

Radix Scutellariae	12 g
Talcum	24 g
Caulis Akebiae	6 g
Poria Cocos	15 g
Polyporus Umbellatus	12 g
Pericarpium Arecae	15 g
Semen Cardamomi Rotundi	6 g

All the above drugs are to be decocted in water for oral administration.

Modification: As same as those in the type of wind – heat in lung meridian.

2. External Treatment

1) Use *Effectual nose drops* for nasal drip, three times a day.

2) Drop nose with 25% *Nose drops of Cortex moutan radicis*, 3 times a day.

3) Use *Nose drops of green Chinese onions* for nasal drip. Take some juice of green *Chinese onions* and have it filtered. Add to it some physiological saline to make a solution of 40%. Drip the solution into the nose, three times a day.

4) Blow into the nose some herbal powder made from the following drugs: 3 grams of *Rhizoma Coptidis*, 3 grams of *Flos Magnoliae* and 0.6 grams of *Borneolum Syntheticum*. Grind these drugs together into fine powder and blow it into the nose, three times a day.

Acupuncture and Moxibustion

1. Acupuncture: Yìntáng(EX − HN3), Yíngxiāng(LI20), Tàiyáng(EX − HN5), Hégǔ(LI4), Fēngchí(GB20), Qūchí(LI11) and Zúsānlǐ(ST36). Each time 2 to 3 acupoints are punctured and manipulated with strong stimulation, and the treatment is given once a day.

2. Auricular Acupuncture: Puncture the head zone in the auricle. It can relieve headache markedly or eliminate headache.

3. Auricular Injection Therapy: It is to inject 0.5 ml of *Yuxingcao injectio* into Fèishū(BL13).

Chapter Seven
Chronic Nasosinusitis

Chronic nasosinusitis, mostly caused by unthorough-going treatment of acute nasosinusitis or by its repeated occurrences, often attacks several nasal sinuses simultaneously. Its clinical features are pus-like nasal discharge and nasal obstruction. It also falls into the category of "Bí yuān" which refers to rhinorrhea with turbid discharge.

ETIOLOGY AND PATHOGENESIS

It is related to deficiency of the lung and spleen which fail to protect the surface and fail to expel pathogenic evils, resulting in rough flow of qi and blood in the nose, and dysfunction in fluid transportation and transformation, which in turn causes accumulation of pathogenic damp and turbidity in the nose, and hence decay as well as suppuration.

MAIN SYMPTOMS AND SIGNS

1. A large volume of lingering, tenacious and white nasal discharge without stinking odor, decrease of smelling ability, intermittent severity of nasal obstruction, nasal obstruction relieved after blowing the nose and aggravated by exposure to wind and cold.

2. Slight red swelling in nasal mucosa, purulent secretion in meatus concha ethmoturbinalis majoris and rhinal fissure.

3. Pale tongue, thin and white tongue coating, soft and slow and feeble pulse.

4. Accompanied by dizziness, distending sensation in the head, bradyphrenia, shortness of breath, lassitude, low voice, reluctance in speaking.

MAIN POINTS OF DIAGNOSIS

1. Much sticky and white or thick and yellow pus – like nasal discharge flows out from the nose, often blown out through the anterior narises or inhaled in through the posterior narises and then spit out.

2. Nasal obstruction is alternate or intermittent, and may be relieved after the nasal discharge is blown out. If polyp is formed the obstruction will be continuous.

3. Osphresis is obtuse.

4. The inferior nasal concha is swollen, with pus – like discharge in the middle nasal meatus and the olfactory cleft. The middle nasal concha may show hypertrophy or polypoid change and polyp may be formed in the middle nasal meatus.

5. **X – ray** photo of the nasal sinuses often shows that the shadows of the cavities of the nasal sinuses have darkened and the mucous membranes thickened, or sign of empyema in the cavities of the sinuses may be present.

6. The patient has a feeling of heaviness, fullness, distending pain and discomfort in the head.

DIFFERENTIATION AND TREATMENT OF COMMON SYNDROMES

1. Internal Treatment

1) the stagnant heat in the lung meridian

Main Symptoms and Signs: There are symptoms such as much yellow turbid nasal discharge, long duration of nasal obstruction, hyposmia, the middle and inferior nasal conchae swollen with empyema or polyp around the former. The accompanying symptoms are dizziness, a sensation of distention in the head and hypomnesia as well. The tongue fur is yellowish and the pulse is taut and thready.

Therapeutic Principles: Clear away pathogenic heat, ventilate the lung and rid turbid nasal discharge to remove obstruction from the upper orifices.

Recipe: *Magnolia flower decoction for purging lung – heat* combining with *Xanthium powder*

Flos Magnoliae	9 g
Rhizoma Anemarrhenae	9 g
Rhizoma Cimicifugae	9 g
Herba Menthae	9 g
Frucus Xanthii	9 g
Fructus Gardeniae	15 g
Radix Ophiopogonis	15 g
Bulbus Lillii	15 g
Folium Eriobotryae	15 g
Radix Astragali seu Hedysari	18 g
Gypsum Fibrosum	30 g
Radix Angelicae Dahuricae	18 g
Radix Glycyrrhizae	6 g

All the above drugs are to be decocted in water for oral administration.

2.) **qi – deficiency of both the lung and spleen**

Main Symptoms and Signs: Much of sticky and white or thick and yellow nasal discharge runs out from the nose. Nasal obstruction is sometimes severe and sometimes relieved. The osphresis is poor. Dizziness, a feeling of distention in the head, shortness of breath, asthenia, cough with white sputum and poor appetite are present. The tongue is light red with thin and white fur on it and the pulse is thready and feeble.

Therapeutic Principles: Tonify and nourish both the lung and spleen and discharge pus to remove obstruction from the upper orifices.

Recipe: *Xanthium powder* combining with *Pill for warming the lung to stop running nose*

Frucus Xanthii	9 g
Flos Magnoliae	9 g
Herba Menthae	9 g
Radix Glycyrrhizae Praeparata	9 g
Fructus Chebulae	9 g
Radix Platycodi	9 g
Otolith Pseudosciaenae	9 g
Radix Ginseng	9 g
Herba Schizonepetae	12 g

Radix Angelicae Dahuricae	18 g
Herba Asari	3 g

All the above drugs are to be decocted in water for oral administration.

Modification: For those with yellow and turbid nasal discharge, add 30 grams of *Herba Taraxaci*, 30 grams of *Flos Lonicerae* and 15 grams of *Herba Houttuyniae*. For those who have loose stool due to deficiency of the spleen, add 30 grams of *Semen Coicis* and 9 grams of *Rhizoma Atractylodis Macrocephalae*. For those with dizziness and a feeling of distention in the head, add 15 grams of *Flos Chrysanthemi* and 9 grams of *Rhizoma Ligustici Chuanxiong*.

3) **qi-deficiency of lung due to pathogenic wind-cold factors**

Therapeutic Principles: Warm and tonify lung-qi for dispersing and expelling wind and cold.

Recipe: *Wen fei tang*

Radix Astragali seu Hedysari	18 g
Rhizoma Cimicifugae	12 g
Radix Puerariae	15 g
Rhizoma seu Radix Notopterygii	9 g
Radix Ledebouriellae	12 g
Herba Ephedrae	3 g
Flos Caryophylli	6 g
Radix Glycyrrhizae	6 g
Caulis Allii Fistulosi	3 stems

All the above drugs are to be decocted in water for oral administration.

Modification: For headache and dizziness, add *Radix Angelicae Dahuricae* 15 g and *Rhizoma Ligustici Chuanxiong* 9 g. For severe nasal obstruction, add *Flos Magnoliae* 9 g and *Frucus Xanthii* 12 g. For yellow and thick nasal discharge complicated by secondary affection of external evils, add *Flos Chrysanthemi* 15 g, *Radix Scutellariae* 12 g and *Radix Platycodi* 12 g.

In cases with obvious spleen qi deficiency, it is advisable to prescribe *Shen ling baizhu wan* modification instead.

Chinese Patent Medicine

Tong xuan li fei wan. Take one pill each time, 3 times a day. *Huo dan wan*. Take 6 g each time, 3 times a day.

2. External Treatment

1) Use *Effectual nose drops* for drip, three times a day.

2) Use *Nasal sinus perfusate for perfusion of nasal sinus*. Its ingredients are as follows:

Radix Astragali seu Hedysari	60 g
Flos Magnoliae	30 g
Radix Angelicae Dahuricae	30 g
Herba Menthae	30 g
Folium Epimedii	30 g
Flos Chrysanthemi Indici	30 g
Ramulus Cinnamomi	30 g
Radix Angelicae Sinensis	30 g

All the above drugs are to be decocted in water twice. Mix the decoction with the distilled liquid which has been recovered during the decocting process. Put q.s. of antiseptic in the mixture and fill ampules with the mixture. Then sterilize it for use. After puncture and irrigation of the maxillary sinus are done, fill it with 2–3 ml of the perfusate. This is done twice a day.

3) Decoct 9 g of *Herba Centipedae* and *Herba Cayratia Japonica* and *Radix Scutellariae* into thick liquor, and then to drop the nose with the filtrated liquor, 3 to 4 times a day.

4) Blow a little *Yu nao shi san* into the nose, twice to three times a day.

Acupuncture and Moxibustion

The main points are **Yíngxiāng**(LI20), **Hégǔ**(LI4), **Shàngxīng**(DU23), and **Bǎihuì**(DU20). The additional points are **Cuánzhú**(BL2), **Yìntáng**(EX – HN3), **Tōngtiān**(BL7) and **Fēngchí**(GB20). The treatment is given once a day. The main acupoints must be used in every treatment and the additional acupoints are chosen alternatively. All the acupoints are manipulated by tonifying technique, and with the needles retained for 10 to 15 minutes. Seven to ten days consisted of one course of treatment.

It is supposed to heat **Qiándǐng**(DU21), **Yíngxiāng**(LI20) and **Shàngxīng**(DU23) with ignited moxa–stick till the patient feels warm and local skin becomes red in color.

In the case with nasal polyp, an operation should be performed to have it removed, and this will be conducive to sinus drainage.

Chapter Eight
Epistaxis

$E_{pistaxis}$ (rhinorrhagia) is a common clinical symptom caused by many reasons and happening in various diseases. In mild cases, only nasal discharge is mixed with blood, and in severe cases it may endanger the patient's life.

ETIOLOGY AND PATHOGENESIS

The most common sites of nasal bleeding are the mucosal vessels over the cartilaginous nasal septum and the anterior tip of the inferior turbinate. Bleeding is usually due to external trauma, nose picking, nasal infection, or drying of the nasal site cannot be seen; these can cause great problems in management. If the blood drains into the pharynx and is swallowed, nosebleed may escape diagnosis. In these cases, bloody vomitus may be the first clue.

Underlying causes of nosebleed such as blood dyscrasia, hypertension, hemorrhagic disease, nasal tumors, and certain infectious diseases (measles or rheumatic fever) must be considered in any case of recurrent or profuse nosebleed without obvious causes.

In traditional Chinese medicine, the condition is termed "Bí nũ", which simply means epistaxis, "Bí hóng" (flood – like nosebleed), "Hóng hàn" (red sweat) and is thought to be caused by dry lungs.

ETIOLOGY AND PATHOGENESIS

The reasons of rhinorrhagia can be listed in the following:
1. **Heat Preponderance:** It indicates hat the invaded pathogenic heat mixes with internal accumulated heat and causes hyperactivity o heat in the lung and

stomach, resulting in crazy circulation of blood;

   2. **Reverse-flowing** qi: For example, frustration and anger turn the stagnation of liver qi into fire which flares and brings blood upwards, pushing blood to circulate outside of vessels;

   3. **Yin Deficiency in the Lung and Kidney**: It refers to flaming-up of deficient fire which injures collaterals in the nose;

   4. **Spleen Qi Deficiency**: It refers to dysfunction of spleen qi which fails to restrain *blood* to circulate inside the blood vessels, causing extravasation. Also there is nasal bleeding due to trauma, which is regarded as syndrome of blood stasis.

MAIN SYMPTOMS AND SIGNS

   1. In mild case, there is bloody nasal discharge or slight nasal bleeding. In severe cases, there is gushing nasal bleeding, very often at sudden onset. The blood can flow out from the anterior nostrils and also can flow into the throat via posterior nasal nostrils. The nasal bleeding can be intermittent, recurrent and continuous and can happen in one nostril and also can happen in both nostrils.

   2. There is capillarectasia or bleeding spots in the anterior part of nasal septum. In severe nasal bleeding, it is not easy to notice bleeding location, and only possible to see gushing bleeding location after cleaning away the blood in the nose. Extensive blood oozing in nasal mucosa can be noticed in recurrent cases.

MAIN POINTS OF DIAGNOSIS

   1. Try to find the spot of nosebleed. Bleeding is apt to occur in the mucous membrane of Kiesselbach's area.

   2. Try to analyze the causes of nosebleed. Detailed inquiry about the history of the case should be made. If possible, examinations of the nasal cavity and nasopharynx, blood text, blood pressure determination, fundus examination and other necessary checks should be done.

   3. The condition depends on the location and the quantity of the nosebleed. Shock may occur in severe cases. Repeated occurrence can cause anemia.

DIFFERENTIATION AND TREATMENT OF COMMON SYNDROMES

1. External Treatment

In the case with active nasal bleeding, it is necessary to stop bleeding first with various hemostatic methods externally in accordance with the principle of "to deal with symptoms in acute condition", and then to identify types of diseases and offer related treatment. The commonly-used hemostatic methods for external treatment are listed as follows.

1) Hemostasis

(1) Cold compress: This is to put towel soaked in cold water or ice-bag on the patient's forehead, neck, or the acupoint **Yǎmén(DU15)**. The neck is the site where *Yangming meridians*, *du channel* and *taiyang meridians* go through, cold compress on the neck is able to restrain *yang*, subside fire for cooling blood and stopping bleeding.

(2) Finger pressing: Insert some aseptic cotton coated with *Powder of puff-ball* or *Yunnan white drug-powder* onto the anteroinferior area of nasal septum, then press the nasal wings with the forefingers to stop the bleeding.

(3) Nose-blowing method: This is to take a little *Crinis Carbonisatus*, *Powder of Lasiosphaera seu Calvatia*, *Baicao shuang*, *Yunnan white powder* and blow into the bleeding location of the nose, several times a day till bleeding stops.

(4) Nose-stuffing method: This is to pound *Herba Agrimoniae*, *Herba Cephalanoploris* and *Herba Ecliptae* to take juice as oral medication, and also able to smash these herbs to stuff the nose.

(5) Plugging: When the above-mentioned methods prove ineffective, the method of plugging either the anterior naris or the posterior naris can be used.

2) Leading Blood Downwards

Repeated occurrence of nosebleed marked by small amount of blood are mostly the result of the injury of blood vessels caused by the upward flow of deficiency-fire. *Powder of Evodia Fruit* can be applied on the sole; or warm water can be used to wash the feet so as to guide the ascending fire downwards; or the paste of *Bulbus Allii* is to be applied onto the acupoint **Yǒngquán(KI1)** which also help to stop the bleeding.

2. Internal Treatment

1) the attack of wind – heat on the lung

Main Symptoms and Signs: Bright – red blood comes out of the nose in drops. There is erosion and oozing of blood at the mucous membrane of the anteroinferior bleeding area of the nasal septum, accompanied with dryness in the nose and mouth, aversion to wind, and fever. The tongue fur is thin and yellow and the pulse floating and rapid.

Therapeutic Principles: Dispel wind, remove heat and cool the *blood* to stop bleeding.

Recipe: *Powder of lonicera and forsythia* with additional drugs

Flos Lonicerae	30 g
Rhizoma Imperatae	30 g
Fructus Forsythiae	15 g
Rhizoma Phragmitis	15 g
Herba Cephalanoploris	15 g
Cacumen Biotae	15 g
Radix Platycodi	9 g
Herba Menthae	9 g
Herba Lophatheri	9 g
Herba Schizonepetae	9 g
Semen Sojae Praeparatum	9 g
Fructus Arctii	9 g
Radix Glycyrrhizae	6 g

All the above drugs are to be decocted in water for oral administration.

2) heat preponderance in lung meridian

Main Symptoms and Signs: Dry nostrils, dry mouth, sore throat, a little nasal bleeding, nasal blood drops or bloody nasal discharge, cough, a little sputum, red tongue, thin and white tongue coating, rapid pulse.

Therapeutic Principles: Expel wind and clarify heat for cooling *blood* and stopping bleeding.

Recipe: *Sang ju yin*

Folium Mori	9 g

Flos Chrysanthemi	15 g
Herba Menthae	9 g
Semen Armeniacae Amarum	9 g
Radix Platycodi	12 g
Fructus Forsythiae	12 g
Rhizoma Phragmitis	15 g

All the above drugs are to be decocted in water for oral administration.

Modification: For profuse bleeding, add *Cortex Moutan Radicis* 12 g, *Rhizoma Imperatae* 15 g and *Fructus Gardeniae* 9 g. For hyperactive heat, add *Radix Scutellariae* 12 g. For swelling and pain in the throat, add *Lasiosphaera seu Calvatia* 3 g and *Radix Scutellariae* 15 g. For yellow and tenacious sputum, add *Fructus Trichosanthis* 18 g, *Bulbus Fritillariae Cirrhosae* 9 g.

Chinese Patent Medicine

Huanglian shang qing wan. Take 6 g each time, 3 times a day. *Sanqi pian*. Take 4 tablets each time, 3 times a day.

3) **hyperactive heat in the stomach**

Main Symptoms and Signs: Profuse and gushing nasal bleeding, dry mouth, foul breath, thirst, preference in drinking water, constipation, yellowish urine, red tongue with yellow coating, full and rapid pulse.

Therapeutic Principles: Clear the stomach and reduce fire for cooling blood and stopping bleeding.

Recipe: *Qing wei tang*

Gypsum Fibrosum	30 g
Radix Scutellariae	15 g
Radix Rehmanniae	15 g
Cortex Moutan Radicis	12 g
Rhizoma Coptidis	9 g
Rhizoma Cimicifugae	9 g

All the above drugs are to be decocted in water for oral administration.

Modification: For profuse bleeding, omit *Rhizoma Phragmitis* 15 g, *Cacumen Biotae* 15 g, and *Herba Ecliptae* 15 g. For constipation, add *Radix et Rhizoma Rhei* 9 g. For swelling and pain in the gums and teeth, add *Rhizoma Anemarrhenae* 12 g.

Recipe: *Decoction of rhinoceros horn and rehmannia* along with *Decoction for clearing away stomach — heat*

Cornu Rhinocerotis	6 g
Cortex Moutan Radicis	15 g
Radix Paeoniae Rubra	15 g
Radix Rehmanniae	15 g
Radix Scutellariae	9 g
Rhizoma Coptidis	9 g
Rhizoma Cimicifugae	9 g
Gypsum Fibrosum	30 g

All the above drugs are to be decocted in water for oral administration except *Cornu Rhinocerotis*, which is to be rubbed with water against the bottom of a bowl and taken after being infused in boiled water.

4) **the flaming — up of liver — fire**

Main Symptoms and Signs: Nosebleed occurs suddenly, with the blood ark red in color and large in quantity, and it comes and goes intermittently. The nasal septum or the posterior part of the nasal meatus bleeds, accompanied by dizziness, headache, dysphoria and irritability, bitter taste and dry throat. The tongue becomes red, with yellow fur, and the pulse is taut and rapid.

Therapeutic Principles: Clear away liver — fire and cool *blood* to stop bleeding.

Recipe: *Decoction of gentian for purging liver — fire with additional ingredients*

Radix Gentianae	9 g
Radix Scutellariae	9 g
Radix Bupleuri	9 g
Caulis Akebiae	9 g
Rhizoma Alismatis	9 g
Fructus Gardeniae	15 g
Radix Angelicae Sinensis	15 g
Semen Plantaginis (decocted after being wrapped in a piece of cloth)	15 g
Herba Agrimoniae	15 g

Rhizoma Imperatae	30 g
Radix Glycyrrhizae	6 g

All the above drugs are to be decocted in water for oral administration.

Modification: For dizziness, omit *Radix Bupleuri* and add *Lignum Aquilariae Resinatum* 9 g and *Haematitum* 12 g. For profuse nasal bleeding, add *Nodus Nelumbinis Rhizomatis* 15 g and *Radix Rubiae* 15 g. For hyperactive heat, add 0.1 g of antelope horn powder and drink with it stirred in boiled water.

5) **yin deficiency of both the live and Kidney**

Main Symptoms and Signs: Light — red blood comes out o the nose in drops, accompanied with dizziness, blurred vision, soreness and weakness of the loins and knees. The tongue is red with thin and white fur on it and the pulse is thready and rapid.

Therapeutic Principles: Nourish and tonify the liver and kidney and replenish *yin* to stop bleeding.

Recipe: *Decoction of Anemarrhea, Phellodendron and Rehmannia with additional ingredients*

Rhizoma Anemarrhenae	9 g
Cortex Phellodendri	9 g
Fructus Corni	9 g
Radix Rehmanniae Praeparata	24 g
Rhizoma Dioscoreae	30 g
Cortex Moutan Radicis	15 g
Rhizoma Alismatis	15 g
Herba Ecliptae	15 g
Colla Corii Asini	15 g
Poria	15 g

All the above drugs are to be decocted in water for oral administration.

Modification: For severe bleeding, add *Nodus Nelumbinis Rhizomatis* 15 g.

Chinese Patent Medicine

Qi ju dihuang wan. Take one pill each time, 3 times a day. *Liuwei dihuang wan*. Take one pill each time, 3 times a day. *Yunnan baiyao*. Take one eighths of the small bottle each time, 3 times a day.

6) **the failure of the spleen to keep the blood flowing within the vessels**

Main Symptoms and Signs: Continuous oozing of light red blood occurs and it may last for a long time. The oozing which covers a large area of the nasal mucosa is accompanied by dim complexion, dizziness, blurred vision, tinnitus and poor appetite. The tongue is light red and the pulse thready and feeble.

Therapeutic Principles: Strengthen the spleen, invigorate *qi*, tonify the *blood* and arrest bleeding.

Recipe: *Decoction for invigorating the spleen and nourishing the heart with additional ingredients*

Rhizoma Atractylodis Macrocephalae	9 g
Arillus Longan	9 g
Radix Ginseng	9 g
Radix Polygalae	9 g
Pollen Typhae	9 g
Radix Astragali seu Hedysari	30 g
Semen Ziziphi Spinosae	18 g
Radix Angelicae Sinensis	15 g
Herba Agrimoniae	15 g
Radix Glycyrrhizae Praeparata	9 g
Radix Aucklandiae	6 g
Colla Corii Asini	6 g
Poria	15 g

All the above drugs are to be decocted in water for oral administration.

Modification: For those with nosebleed due to blood-heat, add 30 grams of *Rhizoma Imperatae*, 30 grams of *Herba Cephalanoploris*, 30 grams of *Cacumen Biotae* and 30 grams of *Gypsum Fibrosum*. For those with nosebleed due to *yin*-deficiency, add 30 grams of *Radix Pseudostellariae*, 15 grams of *Radix Paeoniae Alba*, 15 grams of *Fructus Lycii*, 18 grams of *Herba Agrimoniae* and 15 grams of *Rhizoma Achyranthis Bidentatae*. For those with nosebleed due to *qi*-deficiency, add 6 grams of *Radix Ginseng*, 30 grams of *Radix Astragali seu Hedysari*, 15 grams of *Radix Angelicae Sinensis* and 9 grams of *Crinis Carbonisatus*.

Chinese Patent Medicine

Renshen jian pi wan. Take one pill each time, 3 times a day.

7) epistaxis due to traumata

Main Symptoms and Signs: Bloody oozing due to bruise in the nasal tissue, local swelling and distention in blue and purple color, capable to be accompanied by nasal bone fracture.

Therapeutic Principles: Activate blood and remove stasis for stopping bleeding.

Recipe: *Huo xue zhi tong tang*

Gummi Olibanum	6 g
Pericarpium Citri Reticulatae	12 g
Lignum Sappan	9 g
Flos Carthami	9 g
Radix Notoginseng (powder)	1.0 g
Eupolyphaga seu Steleophaga	9 g
Caulis Cercis Sinensis	9 g
Radix Paeoniae Rubra	15 g
Herba Centella Asiatica	6 g
Radix Angelicae Sinensis	12 g
Rhizoma Ligustici Chuanxiong	9 g

All the above drugs are to be decocted in water for oral administration.

Modification: In the case with injury of qi due to profuse bleeding, it is necessary to prescribe *Du shen tang* immediately in order to benefit qi for rescuing prostration. In the case with poor appetite, it is advisable to take out *Gummi Olibanum* and add 15 g of charred *Fructus Crataegi*.

Chapter Nine
Nasal Vestibulitis

Nasal vestibulitis refers to diffuse inflammation of the skin in nasal vestibulum. In traditional Chinese medicine, it is called "Bí gān" (nasal furuncle) and "Bí chuāng" (nasal boil).

ETIOLOGY AND PATHOGENESIS

It is due to the mixture of invaded wind – heat evils and heat in the lung meridian, or due to dampness of the spleen which steams and fumes the nasal tissues and skin.

MAIN SYMPTOMS AND SIGNS

1. At the initial stage, there are burning heat and dryness in the skin of nasal vestibulum, slight and painful sensation, millet – size papulae.
2. Afterwards, the superficial skin becomes erosive, producing yellowish effusion and scab. The anterior nostrils are often stuffed by scab, disturbing respiration.
3. Gradually, the local skin becomes thick, reddish and rhagadiform. The nasal hairs start to shed and the condition becomes intractable and recurrent.

DIFFERENTIATION AND TREATMENT OF COMMON SYNDROMES

1. **Internal Treatment**

1) **accumulation of heat in the lung meridian**

Main Symptoms and Signs: Burning heat and pain in the skin of the nasal vestibulum, superficial erosion, scanty yellowish effusion, scab, rhagades, occasionally accompanied by headache and fever; crying and scratch on the nose in infants; red tongue, thin and yellow tongue coating, and rapid pulse.

Therapeutic Principles: Clarify heat and resolve toxin; expel wind and assist the lung in dispersing ability.

Recipe: *Huangqin tang*

Radix Scutellariae	12 g
Fructus Gardeniae	9 g
Cortex Moutan Radicis	12 g
Radix Glycyrrhizae	6 g
Fructus Forsythiae	12 g
Herba Menthae	9 g
Herba Schizonepetae	9 g
Radix Paeoniae Rubra	
Radix Ophiopogonis	15 g
Radix Platycodi	9 g

All the above drugs are to be decocted in water for oral administration.

Modification: For severe pain due to excessive accumulation of heat toxin, add *Rhizoma Coptidis* 9 g and *Cortex Moutan Radicis* 12 g. For profuse effusion, omit *Radix Ophiopogonis* and then add *Rhizoma Alismatis* 15 g. For constipation, add *Radix et Rhizoma Rhei* 9 g.

Chinese Patent Medicine

Huanglian shang qing wan. Take 6 g with warm boiled water each time, 3 times a day.

2) **accumulation of spleen dampness**

Main Symptoms and Signs: Redness, swelling and effusion in the skin of the nasal vestibulum, involved nasal wings and lips in severe cases, nasal obstruction, accompanied by abdominal distention and loose stool, thick and greasy tongue with coating, and rolling and rapid pulse.

Therapeutic Principles: Clarify heat dry dampness, resolve toxins and harmonize the stomach.

Recipe: *Decoction for eliminating dampness*

Rhizoma Pinelliae	9 g

Cortex Magnoliae Officinalis	12 g
Rhizoma Atractylodis	9 g
Herba Agastachis	12 g
Pericarpium Citri Reticulatae	12 g
Poria	15 g
Radix Glycyrrhizae	6 g
Rhizoma Zingiberis Recens	3 slices
Fructus Ziziphi Jujubae	6 pieces

All the above drugs are to be decocted in water for oral administration.

Modification: For excessive heat, add *Rhizoma Coptidis* 9 g and *Fructus Forsythiae* 12 g. For profuse effusion due to excessive dampness, add *Talcum* 30 g and *Radix Sophorae Flavescentis* 12 g. For pruritus, add *Radix Ledebouriellae* 12 g and *Cortex Dictamni Radicis* 15 g.

2. External Treatment

1) Add water into the herbal dregs and re-decoct it for warm compress on the nose.

2) To smash *Semen Armeniacae Amarum* and mix it with breast milk for external use.

3) Apply *Qing ge san* on the affected area in those with profuse effusion due to excessive heat.

4) Bake and grind *Herba Orostachyos* into powder for external use in those with lingering erosion.

5) Grind *Cortex Phellodendri* into powder and mix it with yolk oil for external use in those with dry nose and skin rhagades.

Chapter Ten
Rhinopharyngitis

Rhinopharyngitis refers to acute inflammation of the rhinopharyngeal mucosa, characterized by dryness, itching, burning sensation and slight pain in the nasopharynx.

ETIOLOGY AND PATHOGENESIS

It is related to irregular life habit during weather change, in which pathogenic wind and heat happen to attack the rhinopharynx and injure the local mucosa, resulting in the problem.

MAIN SYMPTOMS AND SIGNS

1. Warm sensation, dryness, burning pain and itching in the rhinopharynx and posterior nostrils.
2. Yellowish thick or clotted nasal discharge.
3. Rough respiration due to excretion in the rhinopharynx distending and stuffy sensation in the ear and decrease of the hearing ability caused by the secretion obstructed in the opening of auditory tube.
4. Lack of fluid, lustrousless and dark red color in the mucosa of the rhinopharynx and posterior nostrils, attached with tenacious and purulent secretion.
5. Slight fever in the body, slight thirst, lassitude.
6. Red tongue, thin and white tongue coating, and superficial and rapid pulse.

Chapter Ten

DIFFERENTIATION AND TREATMENT OF COMMON SYNDROMES

1. Internal Treatment

Therapeutic Principles: Expel wind, clear away heat and improve he throat.

Recipe: *Yinqiao san*

Flos Lonicerae	30 g
Fructus Forsythiae	15 g
Radix Platycodi	9 g
Fructus Arctii	9 g
Rhizoma Phragmitis	30 g
Radix Scutellariae	9 g
Frucus Xanthii	9 g
Flos Magnoliae	9 g
Radix Angelicae Dahuricae	18 g
Radix Glycyrrhizae	6 g

All the above drugs are to be decocted in water for oral administration.

Modification: For dryness and thirst in the rhinopharynx, add *Radix Ophiopogonis* 15 g and *Radix Trichosanthis* 30 g. For decrease of hearing ability and tinnitus, add *Fructus Gardeniae* 9 g and *Radix Gentianae* 6 g. For constipation, add *Radix et Rhizoma Rhei* 6 g.

Chinese Patent Medicine

Xi ling jiedu pian. Take 4 tablets each time, twice a day.

Sang ju gan mao pian. Take 4 tablets each time, twice a day.

Bi yan pian. Take 4 tablets each time, twice a day.

2. External Treatment

1) **nasal sniff** Sniff *Bi yuan san*, twice a day.
2) **nasal drip** Drop the nose with *Di bi ling* or *Congbai di bi ye*.

Acupuncture and Moxibustion

Yíngxiāng(LI20), Kǒuhéliáo(LI19), Hégǔ(LI4) and Yìntáng(EX - HN3) are punctured with the needles retained for 20 minutes. The treatment is given once a day.

Chapter Eleven
Nasal Furuncle

Nasal furuncle refers to acute suppurative inflammation happening in sebaceous gland or hair follicle in the nasal vestibulum or nasal tip. It is called "Bí dīng" (nasal furuncle) in traditional Chinese medicine.

ETIOLOGY AND PATHOGENESIS

The pathogenic factors attack and invade through nasal skin and tissue injured in scratching and rubbing the nose. It would be possible to cause the invaded toxins to spread inwards and complicate into septicemia if the healthy energy subsides, resulting in hyperactivity of invaded pathogenic toxins, or there is improper treatment and unsuitable pressure on the nose.

MAIN SYMPTOMS AND SIGNS

1. There are local redness, pain and swelling on the nose, small-size of the boil with its root as deep and hard as a knocked nail, and a yellowish white pus dot on the tip of the boil which breaks spontaneously in one week.
2. It is accompanied by swelling and pain on the lips, face and lower eyelid, fever and constitutional discomfort.
3. In severe cases, there can be high fever, severe headache, serious swelling on the face and nose, restlessness, coma and also possible to endanger life.

MAIN POINTS OF DIAGNOSIS

Clinically it is characterized by:

Nasal Furuncle

1. external millet – size boil, but with its root as hard and deep as a knocked nail,

2. obvious local and constitutional symptoms, and

3. possible tendency of complicating into septicemia, involving ying system and affecting the brain.

DIFFERENTIATION AND TREATMENT OF COMMON SYNDROMES

1. Internal Treatment

1) invasion of exogenous wind – heat toxins

Main Symptoms and Signs: Local redness and swelling on the nose, millet – size boil with its root as hard as a nail, accompanied by redness and swelling on the lips and cheeks, and by non – obvious constitutional symptoms.

Therapeutic Principles: Clarify heat and resolve toxins; expel evils and diminishing swelling.

Recipe: *Wuwei xiaodu yin*

Flos Lonicerae	30 g
Flos Chrysanthemi Indici	15 g
Herba Taraxaci	15 g
Herba Violae	15 g
Radix Semiaquilegiae	12 g

All the above drugs are to be decocted in water for oral administration.

Modification: For superficial syndromes, add *Herba Schizonepetae* 9 g and *Herba Menthae* 9 g.

2) accumulation of internal heat

Main Symptoms and Signs: Yellowish white pus dot on the boil with a high top and soft root, accompanied by fever, headache, and constipation. If the boil breaks and heals spontaneously within one week, it is regarded as a case with favorable prognosis. The tongue is in red color, the tongue coating is yellowish and the pulse is rapid.

Therapeutic Principles: Clarify heat and resolve toxins; reduce fire and diminish swelling.

Recipe: *Huanglian jie du tang*

Rhizoma Coptidis	9 g
Radix Scutellariae	15 g
Cortex Phellodendri	9 g
Fructus Gardeniae	12 g

All the above drugs are to be decocted in water for oral administration.

Modification: For constipation, add *Radix et Rhizoma Rhei* 9 g. For high fever, add *Gypsum Fibrosum* 30 g, *Herba Violae* 15 g. For local redness, swelling and pain, add *Cortex Moutan Radicis* 12 g, *Resina Myrrhae* 9 g. For non-ulcerative suppuration, add *Spina Gleditsiae* 15 g and *Radix Trichosanthis* 30 g. For delayed suppuration due to injury of *qi* and *yin*, add *Radix Astragali seu Hedysari* 18 g.

Chinese Patent Medicine

Niuhuang jie du pian. Take 4 tablets each time, 3 times a day.

Niuhuang shangqing wan. Take one bolus each time, 3 times a day.

3) furunculosis complicated with septicemia

Main Symptoms and Signs: Purplish and dark color in the boil, a dipping boil without suppuration but with a soft and spreading root, serious swelling of the nose, closed eyes, splitting headache, accompanied by high fever, restlessness, nausea, vomiting, coma, delirium, thirst, constipation, dark-red tongue, thick, yellow and dry tongue coating, and flood and rapid pulse.

Therapeutic Principles: Reduce heat and resolve toxins; cool *blood* and open the orifice.

Recipe: *Xijiao dihuang tang*

Radix Paeoniae Rubra	15 g
Radix Rehmanniae	15 g
Cortex Moutan Radicis	15 g
Cornu Rhinocerotis (smashed and taken with water)	6 g

All the above drugs are to be decocted in water for oral administration.

Modification: For severe redness and swelling, add *Radix Trichosanthis* 24 g, *Radix Arnebiae seu Lithospermi* 12 g, *Fructus Gardeniae* 12 g and *Rhizoma Coptidis* 9 g. For coma and delirium, take one pill of *An gong niuhuang wan* in addition. For nausea and vomiting, add *Rhizoma Pinelliae seu Zingiberis* 12 g and *Caulis Bambusae in Taeniam* 12 g. For constipation and injury of *qi* and *yin* due to lingering furunculosis, add *Sheng mai san*.

2. External Treatment

1) Apply *Yulu gao* on boil, once a day.
2) Mix *Sihuang san* with water and apply the mixture on the boil, once a day.
3) Apply *Furong gao* on the boil once a day.
4) Smash 60 grams of *Flos Chrysanthemi Indici* and 60 grams of *Folium Hibisci* for external use, twice a day.

Chapter Twelve
Peripheral Facial Paralysis

Bell's palsy is a paralysis of one side of the face, is facial paralysis which occurs suddenly and mostly after exposure to cold wind or trauma. It may occur at any age but is slightly more common in the age group from 20 to 50. 85 – 90% of the patients get recovered spontaneously. In traditional Chinese medicine, the onset of the illness is thought to be due to derangement of *qi* and *blood* and malnutrition of the channels caused by invasion of the channels and collaterals in the facial region by pathogenic wind – cold or phlegm. If falls into the category of "Zhēn zhòng fēng", "Kǒu yǎn wāi xié" or "Diào xiàn fēng" (deviation of the eye and mouth) in traditional Chinese medicine.

ETIOLOGY AND PATHOGENESIS

It is mostly due to invasion of wind evil into meridians of foot – yangming and hand – taiyang, which results in dysfunctions of meridian *qi* in soothing and distributing abilities, as well as disharmony between ying and wei.

MAIN SYMPTOMS AND SIGNS

1. Sudden onset, peripheral facial paralysis on one side.
2. Dull pain, pressing pain and sensation behind the ear before onset.
3. Progressively, complete or partial facial paralysis, deviation of the mouth and eye, disappearance of nasolabial groove and frontal skin crease, disability of blowing cheeks and of closing the eye.
4. Thin and sticky tongue coating, thready and wiry pulse with rapid speed.

MAIN POINTS OF DIAGNOSIS

1. It often occurs in autumn and winter or between spring and summer, mostly in the middle-aged. The disease usually attacks one side of the face.

2. The diagnosis is based on the symptoms, but most rule out cerebrovascular accidents (strokes) and intracranial tumors. The peripheral facial paralysis patients are specially unable to frown and raise the eyebrow, close the eye of the paralyzed side. The intracranial tumors can be ruled out X-ray examination.

3. The attack comes all of a sudden. At the beginning the patient feels numb at one side of the face, pain around the ear and tenderness in the mastoidal region. Then the mouth becomes wry, the nasolabial groove no longer seen and the facio-buccal region relaxed and powerless. It's impossible to have the cheeks blown up. The eyeballs are still exposed when the eyes are shut. It's difficult to frown and speak. Salivation comes down from the corners of the mouth. The sense of taste is lost but the sense of hearing is hypersensitive. There may be pain in the mastoid region or headache.

DIFFERENTIATION AND TREATMENT OF COMMON SYNDROMES

1. Internal Treatment

1) **the early stage**

Main Symptoms and Signs: The onset is sudden and the duration is short. The mouth and eyes become wry. the eyeballs can always be seen as the eyes can not be closed entirely. There is difficulty in frowning. The accompanying symptoms and signs are headache, discomfort or low fever, red tongue with thin and white fur, and taut and thready pulse.

Therapeutic Principles: Dispelling pathogenic wind and removing obstruction from the channels.

Recipe: Yang-clearing Decoction with additional ingredients

Radix Astragali seu Hedysari	15 g
Radix Angelicae Sinensis	15 g
Fructus Tribuli	15 g

Rhizoma Cimicifugae	9 g
Flos Carthami	9 g
Cortex Phellodendri	9 g
Ramulus Cinnamomi	9 g
Lignum Sappan	9 g
Radix Ledebouriellae	9 g
Periostracum Cicadae	9 g
Radix Puerariae	30 g
Radix Glycyrrhizae	6 g

All the above drugs are to be decocted in water for oral administration.

2) **the late stage**

Main Symptoms and Signs: The course of the disease is protracted. The mouth and the eyes become wry. No wrinkles can be seen on the forehead. The patient has reddish tongue with petechiae on it, thin and white fur, and thready and feeble pulse.

Therapeutic Principles: Promoting qi flow and blood circulation, removing phlegm and clearing away obstruction from the channels.

Recipe: *Powder for Treating Wry - mouth*, compounded with *Decoction Invigorating Yang for Recuperation*

Rhizoma Typhonii	6 g
Scorpio	9 g
Bombyx Batryticatus	9 g
Semen Persicae	9 g
Flos Carthami	9 g
Lumbricus	9 g
Radix Astragali seu Hedysari	30 g
Radix Angelicae Sinensis	15 g
Rhizoma Ligustici Chuanxiong	15 g
Radix Paeoniae Rubra	15 g

All the above drugs are to be decocted in water for oral administration.

For those running low fever, add 30 grams of *isatis root* and 30 grams of *honeysuckle flower*. For those with restlessness due to deficiency and palpitation, add 18 grams of *prepared rehmannia root* and 18 grams of *prepared fleece - flower root* and *suffocation* in the chest and stomach and who are fat and have much sputum, add 6 grams of *arisaema with bile* and 9 grams of *pinellia tuber*.

Another herb therapy is Zhi Jing San Jia Jian

Recipe

Scorpion	2.5 g
Fangfeng	13 g
Larvia of silkworm of rehmannia	10 g
Baifuzi	10 g
Milk veteh	30 g
Radix Angelicae Sinensis	15 g
Unpeeled root of herbaceous peony	15 g
Rhizoma Ligustici Chuanxiong	15 g
Semen Coicis	15 g
Flos Carthami	12 g

All the above herbs make a dose and six to ten doses are prescribed with one dose daily. Each dose is simmered twice and then the broth of each mixed, half of the mixed broth each time, twice a day.

Modification: For pain in the ear and mastoid, add **Caulis Lonicerae** 15 g and **Spica Prunellae** 15 g. For distending pain in eyeballs, add **Semen Cassiae** 9 g and **Semen Celosiae** 9 g. For full and stuffy sensation in the chest and hypochondria, tenacious sputum, add **Caulis Bambusae in Taeniam** 9 g, **Rhizoma Pinelliae**, and **Fructus Trichosanthis**. For slight fever, add **Radix Bupleuri** 15 g and **Radix Isatidis** 30 g.

Chinese Patent Medicine

Qian zheng wan. Take one pill each time with heated wine, twice a day.
Sou feng wan. Take one pill each time with boiled water, twice a day.

Bell's palsy is also divided into the following two types:

1) wind phlegm invasion of collateral

Imprudent living, collateral stroke by wind phlegm, collateral obstruction and blood stagnation, paralysis of facial muscle.

Main Symptoms and Signs: Sudden appearance of mouth deviation and distorted eye, tenderness at **Jiáchē(ST6)**, inability to close eyes, accompanied by chill and fever, numbness of tongue root, thin and white tongue coating, floating and relaxed pulse.

Therapeutic Principles: Expel the wind and resolve phlegm, activate circulation and collateral.

Recipe: *Qianzheng san with additional ingredients*

Pollen Typhae	12 g
Bombyx Batryticatus	12 g
Scorpio	12 g
Radix Angelicae Dahuricae	12 g
Rhizoma Ligustici Chuanxiong	10 g
Scorpio	12 g
Radix Bupleuri	6 g
Smilax Glabra Rhizome	20 g
Periostracum Cicadae	12 g

All the above drugs are to be decocted in water for oral administration.

Modification: For exopahogenic cases, add *Radix Ledebouriellae*, *Herba Schizonepetae*, *Radix Gentianae*, *Radix Puerariae*, *Ramulus Cinnamomi*, *Radix Notoginseng*; associated with wind heat, minus *Radix Angelicae Dahuricae*, add *Herba Menthae*, *Flos Lonicerae*, *Flos Chrysanthemi*; for profuse sputum and salivation, add *Succus Bambusae*, *Rhizoma Pinelliae*.

Chinese Patent Medicine

Xiao huo luo dan. One bolus t.i.d. and *Fufang danshen pian*. 4 tablets t.i.d..

folk prescriptions

1) Blood from living finless eel applied to affected side, once daily.

2) Airsaema tuber suitable dose ground into powder, and mixed with fresh ginger juice applied to affected side, changed once every two days.

2) wind agitation due to blood deficiency

Collateral blockage due to *blood* insufficiency, agitation of asthenic wind.

Main Symptoms and Signs: Wry mouth and distorted eye for long time without recovery; paroxysmal tightness of face, with some twitching. Dizziness and blurred vision, palpitation, insomnia. Red tongue proper with little coating. Thready and rapid pulse.

Therapeutic Principles: Nourish *yin* and *blood* to remove wind and make collateral harmonic.

Recipe: *Si wu tang* with additional drugs

Radix Rehmanniae Praeparata	15 g
Radix Angelicae Sinensis	12 g
Rhizoma Ligustici Chuanxiong	
Radix Paeoniae Rubra	10 g
Radix Paeoniae Alba	10 g
Caulis Spatholobi	15 g
Fructus Trichosanthis	12 g
Bombyx Batryticatus	12 g
Scorpio	10 g

Chinese Patent Medicine

Liu wei dihuang wan, one bolus t.i.d. and *Jixueteng pian*, 5 tablets t.i.d..

2. External Treatment

1) Apply adhesive plaster on the acupoints: Dust 0.5 to 1 gram of the powder of Semen Strychni onto a plaster and then apply the plaster on the acupoint of **Tàiyáng**(EX-HN5), **Xiàguān**(ST7) and **Jiáchē**(ST6) of the affected side (more applicable to the regions with tenderness). Change the plaster every 3 days. If blisters appear on the administered part, extract its fluid after disinfection. Then the blisters will get cured spontaneously.

2) Smear the blood of eel onto the affected region: Smear fresh blood of eel onto the buccal skin of the affected side, and hold the mouth angle of the affected side with a metal hook so as to help cure the facial paralysis. This is to be done once a day.

3) Do local massage on the affected region, several times a day.

Acupuncture and Moxibustion

Points: **Dìcāng**(ST4), **Yìfēng**(SJ17), **Jiáchē**(ST6), **Yángbái**(GB14), **Tàiyáng**(EX-HN5), **Hégǔ**(LI4), **Quánliáo**(SI18) and **Xiàguān**(ST7).

Manipulation: 3 to 5 of the above points are selected for each treatment and the therapy is given once daily. **Dìcāng**(ST4) and **Jiáchē**(ST6) are punctured together with one needle inserted horizontally from **Dìcāng**(ST4) to **Jiáchē**(ST6). The following points can also be added to the formula according to the symptoms:

Fēngchí(GB20) for headache; Fēnglóng(ST40) for profuse sputum; Cuánzhú(BL2) and Sīzhúkōng(SJ23) for difficulty in frowning and raising the eyebrow; Cuánzhú(BL2), jīngmíng(BL1), Tóngzǐliáo(GB1), Yúyāo(EX-HN4) and Sīzhúkōng(SJ23) for incomplete closing of the eyelids; Yíngxiāng(LI20) for difficulty in sniffing; Shuǐgōu(DU26) **for deviation of the philtrum; for inability to show the teeth;** Tīnghuì(GB2) for tinnitus and deafness; Wàngǔ(SI4) for tenderness at the mastoid region; and Tàichōng(LR3) for twitching of the eyelid and the mouth.

Electro-acupuncture Therapy

Main Points: Qianzheng(an extra-point) and Yìfēng(SJ17).

Auxiliary Points: Yángbái(GB14), Tàiyáng(EX-HN5) and Dicang(ST4).

Manipulation: One of the main points and two or three of the auxiliary points are prescribed each time. The main point is connected to the negative pole of the electro-acupuncture machine, and the auxiliary points to the positive pole. The frequency is adjusted to 20 to 30 times per minute with an output which can just cause the muscular twitch on the affected side. The treatment lasts for 15 minutes and is repeated once every other day. Ten times consisted of one course.

The patient can be assured that recovery usually occurs in 2 to 8 weeks (or up to one to two years in older patients). In the vast majority of cases, partial or complete recovery occurs. When recovery is partial, contracture may develop on the paralyzed side. Recurrence on the same or the opposite side is occasionally reported. Acupuncture therapy is very effective for this condition.

Qigong

1. **Self-Treatment by Practicing Qigong**

1) Basic Maneuvers···It is advisable to practice Head and Face Qigong.

2) Auxiliary Maneuvers

Those shedding tears ought to lay emphasis on kneading Yángbái(GB14), Sìbái(ST2).

At the onset stage, the pressing and kneading manipulations applied locally should be light; as for those with a long course of disease, the manipulations should be heavier.

2. External Qi Therapy

1) Basic Maneuvers

(1) Press and knead the acupoints **Yángbái(GB14)**, **Chéngqì(ST1)**, **Sīzhúkōng** **(SJ23)**, **Tóngzǐliáo(GB1)**, **Tīnggōng(SI19)**, **Yìfēng(SJ17)**, **Quánliáo(SI18)**, **Yíngxiāng** **(LI20)**, **Jiáchē(ST6)**, **Fēngchí(GB20)** and **Hégǔ(LI4)**.

(2) Apply the flat-palm form, use the pushing, pulling and leading manipulations to emit qi onto the unilateral paralyzed face, conduct the channel qi from front to back and along the Large Intestine Meridian to the terminals of the upper extremities.

2) Auxiliary Maneuvers

In the anaphase of the paralysis, the additional application of the vibrating and quivering manipulation is advised to provoke the channel qi.

MASSAGE

There will be gradual recovery in on or two weeks after its onset. Manipulation of massage may help the recovery of facial nerves and muscular function and reduce sequelae. During the treatment, stimulus of cold to the face and head should be avoided and the patient should knead the face frequently for enhancing the effectiveness.

1. Method: Pushing with one-finger meditation, digital-pressing, pressing, grasping and kneading.

2. Location of Points: **Hégǔ(LI4)**, **Qūchí(LI11)**, **Xiàguān(ST7)**, **Jiáchē(ST6)**, **Yìfēng(SJ17)**, **Tàiyáng(EX-HN5)**, **jīngmíng(BL1)**, **Sìbái(ST2)**, **Yíngxiāng(LI20)**, **Shuǐgōu(DU26)** and **Dìcāng(ST4)**. 3. Manipulation

1) The doctor stands in front and to the side of the sitting patient and holds the posterolateral part of the head with one hand. Using one-finger meditation pushing or thumb-pressing-kneading, the doctor pushes with the other hand repeatedly from **Yìntáng(EX-HN3)** along the superciliary of the affected side to **Tàiyáng(EX-HN5)** for 2 or 3 times first; then pushes repeatedly from **Yìntáng(EX-HN3)** upwards by way of **Shéntíng(DU24)** to **Bǎihuì(DU20)** also for 2 or 3 times; finally, pushes repeatedly from the middle of the forehead via **Yángbái(GB14)** of the affected part to **Tàiyáng(EX-HN5)** for 2 or 3 times.

2) After that, in the above-mentioned way, the doctor pushes downwards repeatedly from **Yìntáng(EX-HN3)** by way of **jīngmíng(BL1)** of the affected side,

along the side of the nose up to **Yíngxiāng**(LI20) for 2 or 3 times. Then the doctor pushes from **Yíngxiāng**(LI20), along the point of **Sìbái**(ST2), **Quánliáo**(SI18), **Xiàguān**(ST7) and **Jiáchē**(ST6) passing the face, to **Dìcāng**(ST4) at the labial angle.

3) Still in the same way mentioned above, the operator pushes from **Dìcāng**(ST4) to **Shuǐgōu**(DU26) **circling the lips, by way of Chéngjiāng**(RN14), and returns to the starting point. Then the operator pushes along the mandible to **Jiáchē**(ST6). Finally rub and scrub softly the affected side of the face with the palm till local warmth and heat are produced.

In the above-mentioned operations, the movement of the hand should pass at every point with a bit more strength exerted and some stimulating manipulations such as digit-pressing used in combination.

4) The doctor stands to the side of the patient and, with one hand holding his forehead, grasps **Fēngchí**(GB20) and the tendons of the back nape up and down repeatedly for three to five times, finally pushes the point Qiaogong for 30 times.

5) The doctor standing behind the patient, grasps **Jiānjǐng**(GB21) with two hands and in an orderly way presses and kneads **Qūchí**(LI11) and **Hégǔ**(LI4).

4. Course of Treatment: Once a day, six days for one course with an interval of 3 days between two courses.

Chapter
Trigeminal Neuralgia

Trigeminal Neuralgia is more or less included in Tóu fēng tóu tòng (headache caused by attack of the head by pathogenic wind) and Piān tóu tòng in traditional Chinese medicine.

ETIOLOGY AND PATHOGENESIS

Attack of the head by pathogenic wind leads to stagnation of the blood and obstruction of the changed giving rise to pain. Since pathogenic wind is characterized by constant movement and rapid change, the occurrence of this disease is abrupt with intermittent pain.

MAIN POINTS OF DIAGNOSIS

1. It is characterized by paroxysmal burning sensation on the face with severe flash pain accompanied with facial spasm and lacrimation which usually last for few seconds and then relieves spontaneously. The patient feels nothing during interval of attacks.

2. The pain is usually induced by muscular movement of the face ad referred to the lips, ala nasi and jaw.

3. Generally, there is no positive symptoms of nerve system.

4. Clinically, it should be differentiated from toothache, sinusitis and glossopharyngeal neuralgia.

Chapter Thirteen

DIFFERENTIATION AND TREATMENT OF COMMON SYNDROMES

1. Invasion of exogenous pathogenic wind – heat (or wind – fire) in liver meridian

Exuberance of fire of liver meridian with production of wind, the flare up of wind – fire resulting in muscular contracture.

Main Symptoms and Signs: Sudden paroxysmal attack of lightening pain, stabbing or needling or burning over one side of face, continuous for several seconds, as frequent as several times in a minute, or only several times i whole day, accompanied by muscular twitching, congested eyes and lacrimation, saliva flowing out from angle of mouth, vexation and easy to lose temper, deep colored urination and constipation. Even a light touch of the affected side may induce the seizure. Tongue proper red, tongue coat thin and yellow. Pulse taut and rapid.

Therapeutic Principles: Dispel pathogenic wind and heat, remove obstruction from the channel and arrest pain.

Recipe: *Xiong zhi shigao tang*

Rhizoma Ligustici Chuanxiong	20 g
Gypsum Fibrosum	30 g
Flos Chrysanthemi	9 g
Herba Menthae	9 g
Lumbricus	9 g
Fructus Arctii	12 g
Radix Angelicae Dahuricae	12 g
Rhizoma Phragmitis	30 g

All the above drugs are to be decocted in water for oral administration.

Modification: For acute pain with muscle cramp, add *whole scorpion, centipede, batryticated silkworm, earthworm*; for exuberant heat with exhaustion of body fluid, add *Rhizoma Anemarrhenae, Rhizoma Dendrobii, Radix Trichosanthis*; for constipation, oral ulcerations and over tongue, add *Radix et Rhizoma Rhei, Cortex Magnoliae Officinalis,* and *mirabilite*.

Chinese Patent Medicine

Longdan xie gan wan, 10 g t.i.d. or *Niuhuang shang qing wan,* 5 g t.i.d. and *Yuanhu zhi tong pian,* 5 tablets t.i.d..

Equal portions of whole scorpion, centipede and batryticated silkworm

Trigeminal Neuralgia

ground into fine powder, 6 g t.i.d.

Acupuncture and Moxibustion

Points: **Cuánzhú**(BL2), **Yúyāo**(EX – HN4), **Tàiyáng**(EX – HN5), **Yángbái**(GB14), **Jiáchē**(ST6), **Jūliáo**(GB29), **Chéngjiāng**(RN14), **Zhìyīn**(BL67), **Nèitíng**(ST44), **Hégǔ**(LI4), **Wàiguān**(SJ5). All are needled with strong manipulation of reducing technique.

Application of acupuncture in combination with needling points such as **Tīnggōng**(SI19), **Xiàguān**(ST7), **Hégǔ**(LI4), **Sìbái**(ST2), etc. will obtain better result.

2. invasion of exogenous pathogenic wind – cold

Main Symptoms and Signs: Severe pain, aversion to cold, fever, thin and white tongue coating, and wiry and tense pulse.

Therapeutic Principles: Dispel cold and arrest pain.

Recipe: *Chuanxiong cha tiao san*

Rhizoma Ligustici Chuanxiong	30 g
Radix Angelicae Dahuricae	12 g
Rhizoma seu Radix Notopterygii	12 g
Radix Ledebouriellae	12 g
Herba Asari	6 g
Herba Schizonepetae	9 g
Herba Menthae	6 g
Radix Aconiti Kusnezoffii Praeparata	9 g
Radix Glycyrrhizae	6 g

All the above drugs are to be decocted in water for oral administration.

Modification: In case of severe pain or no significant therapeutic effect after taking the above decoction, add *Scolopendra* 6 pieces and *Scorpio* 6 g which are charred by baking and then ground into fine powder to be taken with warm boiled water.

Application of acupuncture in combination with needling points **Tóuwéi**(ST8), **Lièquē**(LU7), **Jiáchē**(ST6), **Xiàguān**(ST7), **Hégǔ**(LI4), etc. may obtain even better result.

3. obstruction of the channel by stasis of blood

Main Symptoms and Signs: Repeated attack of fixed stabbing pain, tinnitus, deafness, dark red tongue with possible stagnant spots, and thready and hesitant pulse.

Therapeutic Principles: Activate *blood* stasis and arrest pain.

Recipe: *Tong qiao zhitong tang* with modification

Rhizoma Ligustici Chuanxiong	30 g
Radix Paeoniae Rubra	15 g
Semen Persicae	15 g
Flos Carthami	9 g
Rhizoma Zingiberis Recens	3 slices
Bulbus Allii	1 decimeter

All the above drugs are to be decocted in water for oral administration.

4. hyperactivity of yang due to yin deficiency

It is due to long standing fire exuberance with exhaustion of *yin* fluid, the kidney water can not nourish the liver, with the upward disturbance of wind *yang*.

Main Symptoms and Signs: Paroxysmal distending hemicrania, contracture of the cranial angle, with referred pain to teeth, witching of facial muscle, dryness of mouth and throat, dysphoria and insomnia, urine scanty in amount and deep colored. Red tongue proper with dry and yellow coating. Taut, thready and rapid pulse.

Therapeutic Principles: Cultivate the kidney and nourish the liver; subdue the liver *yang* and arrest the pain.

Recipe:

Gastrodiae	12 g
Ramulus Uncariae cum Uncis	24 g
Radix Polygoni Multiflori	30 g
Radix Rehmanniae	15 g
Flos Chrysanthemi	12 g
Fructus Trichosanthis	12 g
Periostracum Cicadae	12 g
Scorpio	12 g

All the above drugs are to be decocted in water for oral administration.

Modification: Exuberance of liver-fire, dysphoria and easy to lose temper, plus *Radix Gentianae*, *Fructus Gardeniae*. With prominent insomnia, add *Fructus Jujubae Indici*, *Radix Polygoni Multiflori*. For severe twitching of facial muscle, add *earthworm*, *batryticated silkworm*, *scopion*.

Chinese Patent Medicine

Qu ju dihuang wan. One bolus t.i.d. and *Magnetite powder* 3 g, *Cinnabar powder* 1 g (to be swallowed with water), three times a day.

Acupuncture and Moxibustion

1) Body Points: **Shènshū(BL23)**, **Gānshū(BL18)**, **Hòuxī(SI3)**, **Zúsānlǐ(ST36)**, **Nèitíng(ST44)** (all with reinforcing technique), **Cuánzhú(BL2)**, **Yúyāo(EX-HN4)**, **Tàiyáng(EX-HN5)**, **Yángbái(GB14)**, **Jiáchē(ST6)**, **Chéngjiāng(RN14)** (all reducing method).

Ear Points: Kidney, gallbladder, liver, sympathetic.

Part Two   Laryngopharyngeal Diseases

Chapter One
Acute Pharyngitis

Acute pharyngitis, an acute inflammation of he pharyngeal mucous membrane and the submucous lymphoid tissues, occurs mostly in winter and spring. According to modern medicine, the most common causes are bacterial or viral infection and rarely it is due to inhalation of irritant gases or ingestion of irritant lights. Clinically, it has the following main characteristics: dryness and soreness as well as a sensation of burning in the throat. In traditional Chinese medicine it belongs to the categories of "Hóu bì" (inflammation of the throat) or "Hóu fēng" (acute throat trouble).

ETIOLOGY AND PATHOGENESIS

Due to abnormal climate, unseasonable weather and carelessness about daily life, defense mechanism of the lung becomes so instable that the wind-heat evil takes advantage to attack the throat through the mouth and nose, causing damage of the lung and pathogenic heat to flare up with the result of swelling and pain of the throat. In this way, the disease occurs.

MAIN SYMPTOMS AND SIGNS

1. Pain of the throat, which becomes more severe when swallowing dryly.
2. Fever of 37.5℃ - 39℃, general discomfort, headache, poor appetite and constipation.

3. Diffuse congestion and swelling in the pharynx, particularly in the faux, edema of cion, possible coating on the posterior pharyngeal mucous wall and tonsils with secretion, in most cases, enlargement and tenderness of lymph nodes in the neck.

4. Red, tender tongue with thin, whitish or light yellowish fur, and floating and rapid pulse.

MAIN POINTS OF DIAGNOSIS

1. Dryness, a sensation of burning heat and soreness of the throat are present. When the patient swallows without food, the soreness becomes more severe. Or there may be itching and cough.

2. The patient runs a fever, the temperature ranging in most cases from 37.5℃ - 39℃. The accompanying symptoms of all-over discomfort, headache and nausea may occur.

3. The retropharynx mucous membranes congest diffusively, swell and become bright red. The lymph follicles are red and swollen, with exudates on the retropharynx wall. The lateral pharyngeal bands also show redness and swell. The lymph nodes may be enlarged and have tenderness.

4. The white blood count often increases.

DIFFERENTIATION AND TREATMENT OF COMMON SYNDROMES

1. Internal Treatment

1) the type of wind - heat invasion

Main Symptoms and Signs: Dryness, a sensation of burning heat and soreness in the throat and congestion of the retropharynx wall, or accompanied by fever, headache, itching and cough, nasal obstruction and running nose. The tongue is red with thin and yellow fur on it and the pulse is floating and rapid.

Therapeutic Principles: Disperse pathogenic wind and heat and promote subsidence of swelling to relieve sore throat.

Recipe: *Decoction for treating sore throat*

Flos Lonicerae	18 g
Fructus Forsythiae	15 g
Radix Scrophulariae	15 g
Radix Trichosanthis	15 g
Rhizoma Phragmitis	15 g
Spica Schizonepetae	9 g
Herba Menthae	9 g
Fructus Arctii	9 g
Bombyx Batryticatus	9 g
Radix Peucedani	9 g
Flos Farfarae	9 g
Bulbus Fritillariae Cirrhosae	9 g
Radix Platycodi	6 g
Radix Glycyrrhizae	6 g

All the above drugs are to be decocted in water for oral administration.

Modification: For those with cough, add *Radix Asteris* 12 g. For abundant expectoration, add *Semen Pruni Armeniacae* 6 g. For headache, add *Flos Chrysanthemi* 12 g. For dryness in he pharynx, add *Radix Ophiopogonis* 15 g. For severe pain in the pharynx, add *Rhizoma Belamcandae* 12 g, and *Physalis Alkekengi* 12 g.

Chinese Patent Medicine

Si ji qing pian. Take 3 - 4 tablets, twice a day.

Liu shen wan. Keep 4 - 6 pills in the mouth for sucking, 3 - 4 times a day.

2) **accumulated heat in the lung and stomach**

Main Symptoms and Signs: The patient has a distinct sore throat, difficulty in swallowing, red swollen pharynx and retropharynx lymph follicles with yellow-white specks on the latter, distinctly swollen lateral pharyngeal bands, accompanied by fever, headache and thick sputum. The tongue is red, with thick and yellow fur, and the pulse is taut and rapid.

Therapeutic Principles: Clear away heat and toxin to relieve sore throat.

Recipe: Universal relief decoction for disinfection

Rhizoma Coptidis	9 g
Radix Scutellariae	9 g
Lasiosphaera seu Calvatia	9 g

Fructus Arctii	9 g
Bombyx Batryticatus	9 g
Pericarpium Citri Reticulatae	9 g
Herba Menthae	9 g
Rhizoma Cimicifugae	9 g
Radix Bupleuri	
Radix Isatidis	30 g
Fructus Forsythiae	15 g
Radix Scrophulariae	9 g
Radix Platycodi	6 g
Radix Glycyrrhizae	3 g

All the above drugs are to be decocted in water for oral administration.

Modification: For those with headache, add 15 grams of *Flos Chrysanthemi* and 15 grams of *Folium Mori*. For those with much sputum, add 9 grams of *Rhizoma Belamcandae*, 9 grams of *Concretio Silica Bambusae*, 18 grams of *Fructus Trichosanthis*, and 10 ml *Succus Bambusae*. For those with constipation, add 9 grams o *Radix et Rhizoma Rhei* and 6 grams of *Natrii Sulphas* which is to be taken after being infused in boiling decoction. For those with high fever, add 30 grams of *Gypsum Fibrosum*, 15 grams of *Cortex Moutan Radicis* and 15 grams of *Radix Paeoniae Rubra*.

2. External Treatment

Recipe: *Powder of Borneol and Borax*

Natrii Sulphas Exsiccatus	15 g
Cinnabaris	1.5 g
Borax	9 g
Borneolum Syntheticum	1.5 g

All the above drugs are to be ground together into fine powder and insufflated onto the pharynx, three times a day.

Recipe: *Powder of remains of human urine for treating aphthae*

white remains of human urine	60 g
Catechu	30 g

Cortex Phellodendri	9 g
Indigo Naturalis	9 g
Borneolum Syntheticum	1.5 g
Herba Menthae	6 g

All the above drugs are ground together into fine powder and insufflated onto the pharynx, three or four times a day.

Xi lei san or *Zhu huang san* for local insufflation, 3 - 4 times a day.

Gargles: Decoct the following into 50 ml liquor for gargling, several times a day.

Flos Lonicerae	30 g
Fructus Forsythiae	15 g
Herba Schizonepetae	12 g
Radix Ledebouriellae	12 g
Herba Menthae	6 g
Radix Glycyrrhizae	6 g

Acupuncture and Moxibustion

1) **Acupuncture:** Select **Shàoshāng(LU11)**, **Shāngyáng(LI1)**, **Hégǔ(LI4)** and **Qūzé(PC3)** and use 3 o them each time with reducing technique, once a day.

For fever, use extra acupoints such as **Fēngmén(BL12)**, **Qūchí(LI11)** and **Wàiguān(SJ5)** with reducing technique, once a day.

2) **Injection:** Inject 0.5 - 1 ml liquid of *Yu xing cao zhu she ye* or *Chaihu zhu she ye* at the acupoints **Píshū(BL20)** and **Qūchí(LI11)**, once a day. 3) use shallow puncture for blood letting. Puncture he points of **Shàoshāng(LU11)** and **Shāngyáng(LI1)** with a three - edged needle to let out blood so that pathogenic heat can be removed. Or the reins of the back of the ear are punctured to let out three to five drops of blood. If necessary, the same therapy can be done the next day.

Chapter Two
Chronic Pharyngitis

Chronic pharyngitis, a chronic inflammation o the pharyngeal mucous membrane and submucous lymphoid tissues, is often caused by unthorough – going treatment of acute pharyngitis or repeated occurrences of upper respiratory tract infection and it is related to high – dust environment. Clinically it manifests itself as itching, dryness, soreness of the throat, cough, a feeling of foreign body or obstruction in the throat. It belongs to the category of "Hóu bì" in traditional Chinese medicine.

ETIOLOGY AND PATHOGENESIS

1. sore throat due to yin deficiency

There is general *yin* deficiency in the lung and kidney, or *yin* deficiency of the lung and kidney due to repeated occurrences of pharyngitis by wind and heat, or due to injury of *yin* caused by febrile diseases. With *yin* deficiency in he lung, body fluid is too insufficient to nourish the throat and with *yin* deficiency of the kidney and hyperactivity of fire due to *yin* deficiency, asthenic fire ascends to the throat, resulting in blockage of pharyngeal channels, disorder of *qi* and flaring – up of asthenic fever. In this way, the disease occurs.

2. sore throat due to yang deficiency

There is general *yang* deficiency, or impairment of *yang – qi* due to improper treatment of prolonged illness, or deficient *yin* affecting *yang* due to excessive sexual life, which leads to insufficiency of *yang – qi* and floating of asthenic *yang* up to the throat. In this way, the disease occurs.

MAIN SYMPTOMS AND SIGNS

1. Sensations of a foreign body, itching, burning, dryness and slight pain in

the pharynx.

2. Dark reddish congestion of mucous membrane o the pharynx and slight edema of cion.

MAIN POINTS OF DIAGNOSIS

1. The patient has discomfort, dryness and itching, swelling and soreness, a feeling of foreign body in the throat or being stuck with sputum. He or she often wants to make a slight cough or irritated cough.

2. The patient has a sensation of obstruction and fullness in the throat and a feeling of being blocked when swallowing without any food but no difficulty in eating.

3. The patient is apt to feel nausea and vomiting when he or she gets up in the morning.

4. Examination shows that the mucous membrane of the retropharyngeal wall becomes dark red and congestive, or there are dilatation of micrangium, attachment of exudates, hyperplasia of lymphoid follicles, red swelling and thickening of the lateral pharyngeal bands and pachynsis of the uvula.

DIFFERENTIATION AND TREATMENT OF COMMON SYNDROMES

1. Internal Treatment

1) pharyngitis due to yin deficiency

Main Symptoms and Signs: Sensation of a foreign body in the throat, itching and slight pain in the pharynx, congested dark − reddish mucous membrane o the pharynx on examination, possibly slight fever after lunch, night sweat, feverish sensation in the palms and soles, dry stool or lassitude of the loins and legs, and insomnia due to deficiency, restlessness and dreaminess, little reddish tongue coating, and thin and rapid pulse.

Therapeutic Principles: Nourish *yin* and moisturize the throat; clear away heat and relieve sore throat.

Recipe: *Zhi bai dihuang wan*

Rhizoma Anemarrhenae	9 g
Cortex Phellodendri	9 g
Radix Rehmanniae	12 g
Rhizoma Dioscoreae	15 g
Fructus Lycii	12 g
Cortex Moutan Radicis	9 g
Rhizoma Alismatis	9 g

All the above drugs are to be decocted in water for oral administration.

Recipe: Yang yin qing fei tang

Radix Rehmanniae	12 g
Radix Adenophorae	15 g
Bulbus Fritillariae Cirrhosae	9 g
Cortex Moutan Radicis	9 g
Radix Paeoniae Alba	12 g
Herba Menthae	6 g
Radix Glycyrrhizae	6 g

All the above drugs are to be decocted in water for oral administration.

Modification: For insomnia due to vexation with reddish tongue tip, add *Semen Ziziphi Spinosae* 30 g and *Rhizoma Coptidis* 6 g. For general weakness, uneasy stomach and loose stool, add *Rhizoma Atractylodis Macrocephalae* 9 g and *Poria* 12 g.

Chinese Patent Medicine

Liu wei dihuang wan. Take one bolus, twice a day.

2) pharyngitis due to yang deficiency

Main Symptoms and Signs: Slight pain in the pharynx, dry feeling in the pharynx but with no desire to drink or with a desire for hot drink, pale complexion, low spirit, coldness of hands and feet, clear and watery urine, loose stool, slight redness of the mucous membrane of the pharynx found through examination, light, whitish tongue coating, and deep, thready and weak pulse.

Therapeutic Principles: Warm the kidney and support *yang*, and guide the fire to its origin.

Recipe: Jin gui shen qi tang

Radix Rehmanniae	12 g
Rhizoma Dioscoreae	15 g

Fructus Lycii	15 g
Rhizoma Alismatis	9 g
Cortex Moutan Radicis	9 g
Ramulus Cinnamomi	9 g
Radix Aconiti Praeparata	9 g

All the above drugs are to be decocted in water for oral administration.

Modification: For poor appetite, feeling fatigued and low-spirited, add *Radix Codonopsis Pilosulae* 12 g. For pale lips, dizziness and palpitation, add *Radix Angelicae Sinensis* 12 g, and *Radix Polygoni Multiflori* 12 g.

Chinese Patent Medicine

Jin gui shen qi wan. Take one bolus, twice a day.

3) dryness of the lung due to yin deficiency

Main Symptoms and Signs: There are such symptoms as dryness, slight pain or a sensation o burning heat or foreign body in the throat. Congestion, diffuse dark redness and dilatation of micrangium of the pharyngeal mucous membrane and thickening of the lateral pharyngeal bands may be present, accompanied with itching of the throat, cough with little sputum, fidgets due to deficiency and dreaminess. The tongue is red and the pulse thready and rapid.

Therapeutic Principles: Nourish *yin*, moisten dryness and purge pathogenic fire to relieve sore throat.

Recipe: *Clear dew decoction*

Radix Asparagi	15 g
Radix Ophiopogonis	15 g
Radix Rehmanniae	15 g
Herba Dendrobii	15 g
Folium Eriobotryae	15 g
Radix Rehmanniae Praeparata	18 g
Fructus Aurantii	12 g
Radix Platycodi	9 g

All the above drugs are to be decocted in water for oral administration.

4) stasis of qi and stagnation of phlegm

Main Symptoms and Signs: The patient has a sensation of obstruction or foreign body in the throat, often wants to make a slight cough and feels nausea when getting up in the morning. He may have hyperplasia of lymphoid follicles in the retropharyngeal wall and thickening of the lateral pharyngeal bands, accompanied with chest distress. The tongue is dark red with yellow fur and the pulse thready and slippery.

Therapeutic Principles: Promote circulation of qi, alleviate mental distress and reduce phlegm to resolve masses.

Recipe: *Decoction for clearing the throat*

Folium Raphani	15 g
Folium Eriobotryae	15 g
Radix Scrophulariae	15 g
Rhizoma Belamcandae	9 g
Radix Curcumae	9 g
Semen Oroxyli	9 g
Bulbus Fritillariae Cirrhosae	9 g
Fructus Aurantii	12 g
Flos Trollii	12 g
Oliva	9 g
Radix Trichosanthis	30 g

All the above drugs are to be decocted in water for oral administration.

Modification: For those with poor appetite and loose stool, add 30 grams of *Rhizoma Dioscoreae* and 9 grams of *Rhizoma Atractylodis Macrocephalae*. For those who have soreness and weakness o the loins and feverish sensation in the palms and soles, add 30 grams of *Semen Cuscutae*, 12 grams of *Fructus Corni* and 15 grams of *Rhizoma Cibotii*. For those with symptoms of intense fire due to *yin* deficiency, add 9 grams of *Cortex Moutan Radicis*, 9 grams of *Rhizoma Anemarrhenae*, 9 grams of *Cortex Phellodendri* and 9 grams of *Rhizoma Achyranthis Bidentatae*.

2. External Treatment

1) **Perlingual**.

① Have slices of *Bulbus Lillii* immersed in honey for 7 days, then take them out for perlingual

② Use frosted persimmon for perlingual instead.

③ *Niuhuang yi jin pian*. Keep 2 tablets in the mouth, 3 - 4 times a day.

2) **Oral insufflation of powder drugs**

Bing peng san and *Qing chui kou san* are to be blown onto the pharynx wall.

3) Put the following in hot water and drink it as tea:

Flos Lonicerae	30 g
Fructus Canarii	24 g
Semen Sterculiae Scaphigerae	30 g
Radix Ophiopogonis	30 g

4) Compress on the point **Yǒngquán(KI1)**. Mix *Powder of Evodia fruit* with vnegar for compress on the point **Yǒngquán(KI1)**. Once a day.

Acupuncture and Moxibustion

For sore throat due to *yin* deficiency, select **Fèishū(BL13)**, **Tàixī(KI3)**, **Sānyīnjiāo(SP6)**, **Zúsānlǐ(ST36)**, , **Hégǔ(LI4)**, and **Nèiguān(PC6)** and use 2 - 3 of them, each time with middle or weak stimulation, retaining the needle for 15 - 20 minutes. For pharyngitis due to *yang* deficiency, select **Shènshū(BL23)**, **Píshū(BL20)**, **Zúsānlǐ(ST36)**, **Guānyuán(RN4)**, **Tàixī(KI3)**, **Mìngmén(DU4)**, and **Hégǔ(LI4)** and use 2 - 3 of them, each time with weak stimulation, retaining the needle for 15 - 20 minutes. Alternately, select the above - mentioned points for moxibustion.

Chapter Three
Chronic Hypertrophic Pharyngitis

Chronic hypertrophic pharyngitis refers to a disease with the main symptoms o an increase in the number of the lymphogranules of he posterior pharyngeal mucous wall, hypertrophic lateral bands of the pharynx, sensation of a foreign body, dryness and pains in the throat. In traditional Chinese medicine, it belongs to the category of the asthenia syndrome of "Hóu bì".

ETIOLOGY AND PATHOGENESIS

It occurs after repeated attacks of pharyngitis caused by wind - heat, when the remaining evils in the pharynx cause blockage of he channel passage, stagnation of *qi* and *blood*, and accumulation of sputum and heat; or after years of pharyngitis due to *yin* deficiency, with body fluid turned into phlegm and heat accumulated in the pharynx by constant flaring - up of asthenic *fire*.

MAIN SYMPTOMS AND SIGNS

1. Sensation of a foreign body, dryness and piercing pain in he pharynx.
2. The throat is liable to be irritated, resulting in dry coughing, sickness or vomiting.
3. The pharyngeal mucous membrane is thickened and dark - reddish with its cabolusaries dilated, the lymphogranules on the posterior pharyngeal mucous wall proliferated, and the lateral bands of he pharynx thickened.
4. General weakness, abdominal distention and loose stool.

DIFFERENTIATION AND TREATMENT OF COMMON SYNDROMES

1. Internal Treatment

Therapeutic Principles: Nourish *yin* and clear the lung; promote *qi* circulation and eliminate sputum.

Recipe: *Yang yin qing fei tang*

Radix Rehmanniae	12 g
Radix Ophiopogonis	15 g
Radix Paeoniae Alba	12 g
Cortex Moutan Radicis	9 g
Bulbus Fritillariae Cirrhosae	9 g
Radix Scrophulariae	15 g
Herba Menthae	6 g
Radix Curcumae	9 g
Rhizoma Cyperi	9 g
Fructus Trichosanthis	18 g

All the above drugs are to be decocted in water for oral administration.

Modification: For nausea and vomiting, add *Caulis Bambusae in Taeniam* 9 g. For constipation, add *Fructus Cannabis* 9 g. For obvious increase in the number o the lymphogranules o the posterior pharyngeal mucous wall, add *Bulbus Fritillariae Thunbergii* 9 g and *Radix Scrophulariae* 18 g.

Chinese Patent Medicine

Si ji qing pian. Take 3 – 4 tablets, twice a day.

2. External Treatment

1) *Qing chui kou san* or *Bing peng san*. Insufflate it into the throat, twice to three times a day.

2) *Niuhuang yi jin pian*. Keep 2 tablets in he mouth, 3 – 4 times a day.

3) Cautery: Apply one to three dottings to each of the big ogranales on he posterior pharyngeal mucous wall with heated iron every 3 – 4 days, and stop he cautery as they appear nearly normal.

Chapter Four
Atrophic Pharyngitis

Atrophic pharyngitis refers to a disease with the main symptoms of the pharyngeal mucous membrane becoming atrophic and thinner with the color looking dark − reddish and dim, or the mucous membrane attached with yellowish brown scab. In traditional Chinese medicine, it belongs to the category of "Hóu bi" due to *yin* deficiency.

ETIOLOGY AND PATHOGENESIS

It results from insufficiency of body fluid due to impairment of the liver and kidney, or from body fluid unable to ascend to the pharynx for lack of digesting source due to weakness in the spleen and stomach; or from prolonged irritations by powder and dust, chemical gas, or radiotherapy or surgical operations.

MAIN SYMPTOMS AND SIGNS

1. it usually occurs in the middle − aged or the old.
2. Feeling of dryness, a foreign body in the throat, and frequent vomiturition with frequent sound in the throat and foul breath.
3. The pharyngeal mucous membrane looks dark − reddish, dry and dim, oil − paper alike, possibly attached with dark − yellow crust.
4. Red, tender tongue with thin, whitish or light yellow fur, and thready and taut pulse.

DIFFERENTIATION AND TREATMENT OF COMMON SYNDROMES

1. Internal Treatment

Therapeutic Principles: Nourish *yin* and moisturize dryness; expel heat and relieve sore throat.

Recipe: *Qing zap jiu fei tang*

Folium Mori	9 g
Gypsum Fibrosum	18 g
Fructus Cannabis	9 g
Radix Ophiopogonis	15 g
Semen Dolichoris Album	12 g
Radix Trichosanthis	15 g
Radix Adenophorae Strictae	15 g
Radix Glycyrrhizae	6 g

All the above drugs are to be decocted in water for oral administration.

Modification: For abundant expectoration, add *Radix Astragali seu Hedysari* 15 g, *Rhizoma Dioscoreae* 18 g. For feeling dizzy with pale lips, add *Radix Polygoni Multiflori* 9 g and *Radix Angelicae Sinensis* 12 g.

Chinese Patent Medicine

Niuhuang yi jin pian. 3 – 4 tablets, twice a day.

Run hou wan. Keep 8 pills in the mouth 3 – 4 times a day.

Qing yan wu hua ye. Inhale 10 – 20 ml of it, once a day.

Put the following in hot water and drink it as tea:

Flos Lonicerae	30 g
Semen Sterculiae	30 g
Fructus Canarii	30 g
Radix Ophiopogonis	30 g

Chapter Five
Submucous Hematoma of Pharynx

Submucous hematoma of pharynx refers to sudden bleeding in he soft palate and uvula due to hasty intake of dry food. According to the different locations, hemorrhage happening in uvula is called "xuan qi feng" (hematoma of uvula) and in upper palate, called "fei yang hou" (hematoma of uvula in traditional Chinese medicine.

ETIOLOGY AND PATHOGENESIS

It is related to over intake of spicy and greasy food which causes accumulation of heat in the spleen and stomach, and progressively the long − term accumulated heat turns into fire, burning and damaging the meridians, and hence extravasation; or related to intake of dry food which rubs and injures the meridians, resulting in the problem.

MAIN SYMPTOMS AND SIGNS

1. Sudden purplish and blood blister under the mucosa of uvula or soft palate after dry food intake.
2. Severe sore throat after rupture of a blood blister, aggravated by speaking and swallowing.

DIFFERENTIATION AND TREATMENT OF COMMON SYNDROMES

1. Internal Treatment

Therapeutic Principles: Clear away heat and dissolve toxin for cooling blood and improving the throat.

Recipe: *Huanglian jie du tang*

Rhizoma Coptidis	9 g
Cortex Phellodendri	9 g
Radix Scutellariae	9 g
Fructus Gardeniae	12 g
Radix Scrophulariae	15 g
Cortex Moutan Radicis	12 g

All the above drugs are to be decocted in water for oral administration.

Modification: For severe pain, add *Radix Paeoniae Rubra* 12 g. For constipation, add *Radix et Rhizoma Rhei* 6 g and *Natrii Sulphas* 9 g. For yellowish urine, add *Folium Bambusae* 9 g and *Semen Plantaginis* 12 g.

Chinese Patent Medicine

Huanglian shang qing wan. Take 6 g each time, twice a day.

Niuhuang jie du pian. Take 3 to 4 tablets each time, twice a day.

2. External Treatment

1) **puncture**

Pierce the blister for releasing blood with a sterilized needle in the initial time of the blister.

2) **mouth rinsing**

Decoct in water 15 g of *Flos Lonicerae*, 12 g of *Radix Rehmanniae* and 12 g of *Radix Scutellariae* into 500 ml of liquor with which to rinse the mouth several times a day.

3) **drug – blowing therapy**

Blow *Qing chui kou san* or *Xi lei san* into he throat, 3 to 4 times a day.

Chapter Six
Acute Epiglottitis

*A*cute epiglottitis is characterized by sudden onset, fast progress and easy invasion upon the throat area, and difficulty in breathing. Usually, it is due to accumulation of wind — heat evil and toxins in the epiglottis with the main symptoms of pain in swallowing, redness and swelling of the epiglottis or even with suppuration, which causes obstruction of breathing. In traditional Chinese medicine, it belongs to the category of "Yān yí tòng" (pain in the throat), "Hóu bì" (sore throat) and "é fēng" (sudden obstruction of the throat).

ETIOLOGY AND PATHOGENESIS

The epiglottis, as belonging to the lung system, is the gateway for water, foodstuff and breathing air to come in and go out. Invasion of wind — heat from superficies to interior, or accumulation of heat in the lung and stomach due to addiction to fatty diet causes both the internal and external heat to stagnate in the epiglottis. If the toxic heat is excessive, the epiglottis will go rotting and suppurating.

MAIN SYMPTOMS AND SIGNS

1. Sudden occurrence of sore throat, which becomes severe in swallowing and progresses fast, even with the result of difficulty in swallowing and stagnation of secretion.
2. Vague voice, shortness of breath or even difficulty in breathing.
3. The epiglottis is red and swollen, or pale and swollen like a ball. In a severe case, it is covered with yellow and white pus dots with local parts bulged brightly. The laterocervical lymph nodes become enlarged.
4. Headache, aversion to cold, and high fever possibly as high as 40℃.

… Chapter Six

DIFFERENTIATION AND TREATMENT OF COMMON SYNDROMES

1. Internal Treatment

1. invasion of wind - heat evil into the throat

Main Symptoms and Signs: Aversion to cold, fever, pain in swallowing, fast progress from bad to worse, difficulty in breathing, thin and yellowish tongue coating, and floating and rapid pulse.

Therapeutic Principles: Expel wind and clear away heat; remove toxic substances and promote subsidence of swelling.

Recipe: *Yinqiao san*

Flos Lonicerae	18 g
Fructus Forsythiae	15 g
Cortex Moutan Radicis	9 g
Rhizoma Phragmitis	15 g
Fructus Arctii	9 g
Spica Schizonepetae	9 g
Herba Lophatheri	9 g
Herba Menthae	9 g
Radix Glycyrrhizae	6 g
Radix Platycodi	6 g
Fructus Gardeniae	15 g

All the above drugs are to be decocted in water for oral administration.

Modification: For excessive heat, add *Folium Isatidis* 15 g, *Herba Taraxaci* 15 g. For headache, add *Flos Chrysanthemi* 15 g and *Radix Angelicae Dahuricae* 15 g.

2) excessive heat evil

Main Symptoms and Signs: Severe pain of the throat, difficulty in eating soup and drinking water, vague voice, disturbed breathing into intolerance to cold, fever, thirst, halitosis, constipation, dark - yellowish urine, red tongue with thick yellowish fur, and strong and rapid pulse.

Therapeutic Principles: Clarify heat and remove toxins; disperse *blood* stasis and eliminate pus.

Recipe: *Wu wei xiao du yin*

Flos Lonicerae	30 g
Flos Chrysanthemi Indici	15 g
Herba Taraxaci	30 g
Herba Violae	18 g
Herba Senecio Nudicaulis	15 g
Fructus Forsythiae	15 g
Radix Isatidis	30 g
Bombyx Batryticatus	9 g
Spina Gleditsiae	9 g

All the above drugs are to be decocted in water for oral administration.

Modification: For severe pain and thick sputum, add *Succus Bambusae* 30 ml and *Radix Paeoniae Rubra* 15 g. For constipation and dark-yellowish urine, add *Radix et Rhizoma Rhei* 9 g, *Caulis Akebiae* 6 g. For abscess broken with pus running out, omit *Radix Scutellariae* and add *Radix Trichosanthis* 30 g.

Chinese Patent Medicine

Qing yan li ge wan. Take one or two boluses with warm water, twice a day.

Liu shen wan. Keep 10 pills in the mouth and then swallow slowly after they are dissolved.

Huanglian shang qing wan. Take 6 g of it twice a day.

Recipe:

Cortex Moutan Radicis	15 g
Fructus Gardeniae	15 g
Radix Curcumae	9 g
Rhizoma Belamcandae	9 g

Decocted into liquor and drunk at a draft.

2. External Treatment

1) *Chui hou san* or *Bing huang san*. Insufflate he powder in the throat in the

initial period, twice to three times a day.

2) Cut through and drain the pus out in case of pus formation.

Acupuncture and Moxibustion

1) **Shallow puncture with blood out**: Select and use the points **Shàoshāng** (LU11) and **Shāngyáng** (LI1) in order to purge the heat. Repeat the therapy the second day.

2) **Acupuncture**: Select the points **Hégǔ** (LI4), **Tiāntū** (RN22) and **Qūchí** (LI11) and use two of them each time with strong stimulation, once a day.

3) **Auricular Therapy**: Select corresponding points, use 2 - 3 of them alternatively each time, once a day.

Chapter Seven
Acute Tonsillitis

Acute tonsillitis is an acute nonspecific inflammation of the palatal tonsillae. Its clinical features are fever, headache, sore throat which is aggravated when swallowing, and reddened and swollen palatal tonsillae. It is called "Fēng rè rŭ é" or "é fēng", both referring to acute tonsillitis caused by pathogenic wind-heat.

ETIOLOGY AND PATHOGENESIS

It is related to pathogenic wind and heat which invade through the mouth and nose to attack the lung and stomach, resulting in the condition that heat in the lung ascends and attacks the throat by the lung meridian; or related to accumulation of heat in the stomach and spleen due to preference for spicy and greasy food and further attack of pathogenic wind and heat, resulting in accumulated heat in the throat.

MAIN SYMPTOMS AND SIGNS

1. Fever around 40℃.
2. Sore throat aggravated by swallow, even difficulty in swallow, pain radiating to the ear.
3. Redness and swelling in tonsil, purulent secretion in the opening of crypt, congestion in pharyngeal mucosa, submaxillary lymphadenovarix with tenderness.

MAIN POINTS OF DIAGNOSIS

1. The patient shivers with fever (the highest temperature may be around

40℃) and has accompanying headache and soreness o the limbs. In infant patient convulsion may present.

2. Sore throat occurs and it may radiate to the ears. The pain becomes more severe when the patient swallows and there is even dysphagia in severe cases.

3. The palatal tonsils congest and swell or there may be yellow - white exudate on the lacunae, which in severe cases forms a false membrane that can be easily erased.

4. There may be congestion of the throat as well as redness and swelling of or small white dots on the retropharyngeal lymph follicles.

5. There may be swelling and tenderness of the lymph nodes in the angle of mandible.

6. There is an increase in the number of the white blood cells and neutrophils.

7. The onset is abrupt and its duration is short. Generally it can get cured in 5 - 7 days.

DIFFERENTIATION AND TREATMENT OF COMMON SYNDROMES

1. Internal Treatment

1) **wind - heat type**

Main Symptoms and Signs: They are fever, aversion to col, headache, sore throat, redness and swelling in or yellow - white pus dots on the palatal tonsils, or accompanied with soreness of limbs. The tongue is red with yellow fur and the pulse floating and rapid.

Therapeutic Principles: Dispersing pathogenic wind, clearing away pathogenic heat and removing toxin to subdue swelling.

Recipe: *Decoction for treating tonsillitis*

Herba Schizonepetae	9 g
Radix Ledebouriellae	9 g
Flos Chrysanthemi	15 g
Fructus Forsythiae	15 g
Cortex Moutan Radicis	15 g

Radix Scrophulariae	15 g
Flos Lonicerae	30 g
Gypsum Fibrosum	30 g
Fructus Arctii	9 g
Rhizoma Belamcandae	9 g
Radix Isatidis	45 g
Radix Trichosanthis	18 g
Radix Glycyrrhizae	6 g

All the above drugs are to be decocted in water for oral administration.

Recipe: *Shu feng qi re tang*

Herba Schizonepetae	9 g
Radix Ledebouriellae	9 g
Flos Lonicerae	30 g
Fructus Forsythiae	15 g
Radix Scutellariae	12 g
Radix Paeoniae Rubra	9 g
Radix Scrophulariae	12 g
Bulbus Fritillariae Thunbergii	9 g
Radix Trichosanthis	15 g
Radix Platycodi	6 g
Radix Glycyrrhizae	6 g

All the above drugs are to be decocted in water for oral administration.

Modification: For obvious redness and swelling in tonsil, add *Cortex Moutan Radicis* 12 g. For constipation, add *Radix et Rhizoma Rhei* 6 g, *Natrii Sulphas* 6 g. For foul breath, add *Gypsum Fibrosum* 15 g.

Chinese Patent Medicine

Xi ling jie du pian. Take 4 tablets each tim, twice a day.

Si ji qing pian. Take 3 to 4 tablets each time, twice a day.

Kang yan ling. Take 3 to 4 tablets each time, twice a day.

2) **phlegm – heat type**

Main Symptoms and Signs: High fever, thirst, severe sore throat, difficulty in swallow, foul breath, redness and swelling in tonsil, yellow and white doted effusion or pseudomembrane in the opening of crypt, congestion in pharyngeal mucosa, submaxillary lymphadenovarix with tenderness, red tongue, yellow and sticky tongue coating, rolling and rapid pulse.

Therapeutic Principles: Reduce heat and dissolve toxin for eliminating swelling and improving the throat.

Recipe: *Qing yan li ge tang*

Radix Scutellariae	9 g
Radix Ledebouriellae	9 g
Herba Menthae	6 g
Fructus Gardeniae	9 g
Radix Scutellariae	9 g
Fructus Forsythiae	15 g
Flos Lonicerae	30 g
Rhizoma Corydalis	9 g
Fructus Arctii	9 g
Radix Scrophulariae	12 g
Radix et Rhizoma Rhei	6 g
Natrii Sulphas 9 g	
Radix Glycyrrhizae	

All the above drugs are to be decocted in water for oral administration.

Modification: for yellow and tenacious sputum, add *Fructus Trichosanthis* 18 g and *Bulbus Fritillariae Cirrhosae* 6 g. For high fever, add *Gypsum Fibrosum* 30 g and *Concretio Siliceae Bambusae* 9 g.

Chinese Patent Medicine

Niuhuang jie du pian. Take 3 to 4 tablets each time, twice a day.

Huanglian shang qing wan. Take 6 grams.

2. External Treatment

1) **herbal gargle**

Herba Schizonepetae	4.5 g
Radix Ledebouriellae	4.5 g
Radix Glycyrrhizae	4.5 g
Flos Lonicerae	15 g
Fructus Forsythiae	15 g
Herba Menthae	3 g

All the above drugs are to be decocted in water. The decoction is to be filtered and used as a gargle.

Another recipe for rinsing is as follows:

Flos Lonicerae	30 g
Radix Platycodi	9 g
Radix Scutellariae	12 g
Radix Glycyrrhizae	6 g

Make 500 ml of liquor to rinse the mouth several times a day.

2) **oral insufflation of indigotic powder**

Gypsum Fibrosum	9 g
Indigo Naturalis	3 g
Mentholum	0.15 g
Cortex Phellodendri	0.2 g
Borax	9 g
Borneolum	3 g

All the above drugs are to be ground together into fine powder and put into bottles for use. The powder is to be insufflated onto the pharynx several times a day.

3) **spray inhalation**

In hale 10 to 20 ml of *Qing yan wu hua ye*. Once a day.

Acupuncture and Moxibustion

1) Choose 2 to 3 points each time from **Hégǔ(LI4)**, **Nèitíng(ST44)**, **Qūchí(LI11)** and **Yújì(LU10)** and puncture with reducing method twice a day.

2) Use shallow puncture for blood letting. Puncture the points of **Shàoshāng(LU11)** and **Shāngyáng(LI1)** with a three-edged needle to let out blood so that pathogenic heat can be removed. Or the veins of the back of the ear are punctured to let out three to five drops of blood. If necessary, the same can be done the next day.

3) It is advisable to inject 0.5 to 1.0 ml of *Yuxingcao zhu she ye* or *Chaihu zhu she ye* into both **Píshū(BL20)** and **Qūchí(LI11)**, and the injection is given once a day.

Chapter Eight
Peritonsillar Abscess

P*eritonsillar abscess* refers to acute purulent inflammation in peritonsillar spaces, characterized by fever, sore throat and difficulty in opening the mouth. It belongs to the category of "Hóu yōng" (throat abscess) in traditional Chinese medicine. it is also called "Hóu guǎn yōng" (peritonsillar abscess) or "Qì guǎn yōng" (peritonsillar suppuration) according to the different location.

ETIOLOGY AND PATHOGENESIS

It is related to the long – term accumulation of heat in the spleen and stomach, and secondary infection o pathogenic wind and heat which induce the accumulated heat in the spleen and stomach to ascend and steam the throat, leading to hyperactivity of heat which is condensed into carbuncle.

MAIN SYMPTOMS AND SIGNS

1. Fever over 39℃.
2. Severe sore throat, difficulty in swallowing, salivation.
3. Reflex ear pain on the sick side.
4. Difficulty in opening the mouth.
5. Congestion and swelling in the throat, obvious congestion and prominence in the upper part of arcus glossopalatinus and arcus palatini on the sick side, redness and swelling in tonsil and uvula, motor impairment of the neck, submaxillary lymphadenovarix.

DIFFERENTIATION AND TREATMENT OF COMMON SYNDROMES

1. Internal Treatment

1) the initial stage

Main Symptoms and Signs: Sore throat aggravated in swallow, fever, aversion to cold, headache, peritonsillar redness and swelling to a hard touch, red tongue, thin–white or thin–yellow tongue coating, superficial and rapid pulse.

Therapeutic Principles: Expel wind and clarify heat for eliminating swelling and stopping pain.

Recipe: *Wu wei xiao du yin*

Flos Lonicerae	30 g
Fructus Forsythiae	15 g
Herba Violae	15 g
Herba Taraxaci	30 g
Radix Platycodi	9 g
Herba Schizonepetae	9 g
Radix Angelicae Dahuricae	12 g
Radix Ledebouriellae	9 g
Flos Chrysanthemi	9 g

All the above drugs are to be decocted in water for oral administration.

Modification: For headache, add *Folium Mori* 9 g. For joint pain, add *Ramulus Mori* 15 g.

2) the suppurating stage

Main Symptoms and Signs: High fever, severe sore throat, difficulty in opening mouth, foul breath, headache, stuffy chest, abdominal distention, constipation, yellow urine, redness, swelling and prominence on the acarus palatini on the sick side with a moving touch, motor impairment of the neck, submaxillary lymphadenovarix, red tongue, yellow and sticky tongue coating, rolling and rapid pulse.

Therapeutic Principles: Clarify heat and dissolve toxin for activating *blood* and eliminating swelling.

Recipe: *Qing yan li ge tang*

Flos Lonicerae	30 g
Fructus Forsythiae	15 g
Fructus Gardeniae	9 g
Radix Scutellariae	9 g
Fructus Arctii	9 g
Herba Menthae	6 g
Radix Ledebouriellae	9 g
Herba Schizonepetae	9 g
Natrii Sulphas 6 g	
Radix Scrophulariae	30 g
Radix et Rhizoma Rhei	6 g

All the above drugs are to be decocted in water for oral administration.

Modification: For obvious distending pain in the throat with a moving touch, add *Cortex Moutan Radicis* 9 g and *Radix Arnebiae seu Lithospermi* 9 g. For yellow urine, add *Talcum* 30 g and *Semen Plantaginis* 12 g. For submaxillary lymphadenovarix, add *Spica Prunellae* 15 g and *Herba Violae* 15 g.

Chinese Patent Medicine

Si ji qing pian. Take 4 tablets each time, twice a day.

Huanglian shang qing wan. Take 6 g each time, twice a day.

Niuhuang jie du pian. Take 3 to 4 tablets each time, twice a day.

2. External Treatment

1) **drug - blowing therapy**

Use *Qing chui kou san* or *Bing peng san*, 3 to 4 times a day.

2) **mouth rinsing**

Decoct 4.5 g of *Radix Ledebouriellae*, 4.5 g of *Herba Schizonepetae*, 4.5 g of *Radix Glycyrrhizae*, 15 g of *Flos Lonicerae*, 15 g of *Fructus Forsythiae* and 3 g of *Herba Menthae* into 500 ml of liquor. Rinse the mouth several times a day.

3) **submaxillary lymphadenovarix**

Apply *Fu rong gao* or *Zi jin ding* externally.

Abscess

Incise or pierce abscess or releasing pus.

Acupuncture and Moxibustion

It is advisable to prick **Shàoshāng(LU11)** and **Shāngyáng(LI1)** for bleeding o several drops.

Auricular points such as throat, hear, ear – shenmen, endocrine and adrenal with twisting manipulation, and with the needles retained for 20 to 30 minutes each time.

Chapter Nine
Pharyngeal Paraesthesia

Pharyngeal paraesthesia refers to a functional disease with the main symptoms of various abnormal feelings or illusions of the pharynx such as feeling stuffed by a ball, pressed, itching, sticking, or resistance to swallowing but actually with no difficulty of doing so. In traditional Chinese medicine, it is called "Méi hé qì" (globus hystericus).

ETIOLOGY AND PATHOGENESIS

Depression of seven modes of emotions and stagnation of the liver - qi result in dysfunction of qi incoordination between qi and *blood*, transverse invasion of the spleen by the liver - qi and dysfunction of the spleen in transport, which lead to production of phlegm - dampness and adverse rising of phlegm - qi and its accumulation in the throat. In this way the disease occurs.

MAIN SYMPTOMS AND SIGNS

1. It usually occurs in the female.
2. There is a sensation of a foreign body in the pharynx, such as that of ball - stuffing, itching, compressing, sticking, burning, or obstruction of swallowing yet with no actual trouble.
3. Pharyngeal examination finds nothing abnormal.
4. Mental distress, insomnia, hypochondriac distention, poor appetite and loose stool.
5. Darkish and dim tongue coating and taut pulse.

Pharyngeal Paraesthesia

DIFFERENTIATION AND TREATMENT OF COMMON SYNDROMES

1. Internal Treatment

Therapeutic Principles: Disperse the depressed liver qi, promote qi circulation and resolve the stagnation.

Recipe: *Banxia houpo tang*

Rhizoma Pinelliae	9 g
Cortex Magnoliae Officinalis	12 g
Caulis Perillae	12 g
Poria	15 g
Rhizoma Zingiberis Recens	3 slices

All the above drugs are to be decocted in water for oral administration.

Modification: For hypochondriac pain, add *Rhizoma Corydalis* 9 g. For insomnia, add *Cortex Albiziae* 12 g and for poor appetite, *Fructus Crataegi* 12 g is added.

Chinese Patent Medicine

Xiao yao wan. Take 6 g of it each time, twice a day.

2. External Treatment

Qing chui kou san or *Bing peng san*. Insufflate the powder in the throat, 3 – 4 times a day.

Acupuncture and Moxibustion

Select **Nèiguān(PC6)**, **Hégǔ(LI4)**, **Tàichōng(LR3)**, **Fēnglóng(ST40)**, and use all of them. Retain the needle for 20 minutes, once a day.

Chapter Ten
Acute Laryngitis

Acute laryngitis is an acute inflammation of the laryngeal mucous membranes. If it occurs in infants, the condition will be a sever one. Its clinical characteristics are hoarseness or cough and fever as well as dyspnea in severe cases. In traditional Chinese medicine it belongs to the category of "Bào yīn" (sudden loss of voice), "Jí hóu yīn" (acute aphonia due to throat disease), "Hóu bì" (sore throat).

ETIOLOGY AND PATHOGENESIS

Invasion of the evils of wind — cold or wind — heat into the throat leads to impairment of the lung's dispersing and descending function, incoordination of *qi* and *blood*, stagnation of profuse sputum, and dysfunction of the glottis. In this way the disease occurs.

MAIN SYMPTOMS AND SIGNS

1. Low and hoarse voice; even losing the voice in a severe case.
2. Uneasiness and pain of the throat, severe pain in speaking.
3. Fever, headache and coughing with white — yellowish sputum coming out.
4. Congestion of the faux, congestion and swelling o the vocal cord, unclose of the glottis, congestion of the ventricular bands, and redness and swelling of the arytenoid area even with yellowish pus dots.

MAIN POINTS OF DIAGNOSIS

Acute Laryngitis

1. The patient's voice is low and hoarse or even lost in severe cases.

2. The patient has in the throat dryness, a feeling of burning heat, itching which causes cough, laryngeal pain and occasionally dyspnea.

3. Redness and swelling are present in the vocal cords, aryepiglottic folds and ventricular bands. There is diffusive redness and swelling throughout the laryngeal mucous membrane with exudates attached.

4. The glottis cannot get completely closed.

5. Fever and headache or only low fever may be present.

DIFFERENTIATION AND TREATMENT OF COMMON SYNDROMES

1. Internal Treatment

1) invasion of wind – heat evil into the throat

Main Symptoms and Signs: Sudden hoarseness of voice, itching in the larynx, coughing with little thin sputum, light redness and edema of the ventricular bands, together with intolerance to wind, slight fever, clear and watery nasal discharge, thin and whitish tongue coating, and floating pulse.

Therapeutic Principles: Expel wind and clear away cold; assist the lung in dispersing ability and easing up the voice.

Recipe: *San ao tang*

Herba Ephedrae	9 g
Semen Pruni Armeniacae	9 g
Radix Glycyrrhizae	6 g
Lignum Sappan	9 g
Periostracum Cicadae	9 g
Semen Sterculiae Scaphigerae	9 g
Radix Platycodi	6 g

All the above drugs are to be decocted in water for oral administration.

Modification: For obvious edema o the vocal cod, add *Herba Asari* 3 g. For much itching in the throat and coughing with productive sputum, add *Rhizoma Belamcandae* 9 g, *Radix Asteris* 15 g and *Flos Farfarae* 15 g. For excessive heat, reduce the dosage of *Herba Ephedrae* to 6 g and add *Flos Lonicerae* 30 g.

Recipe: *Decoction of six drugs*

Herba Schizonepetae	12 g
Radix Ledebouriellae	9 g
Radix Platycodi	9 g
Herba Menthae	9 g
Bombyx Batryticatus	9 g
Radix Glycyrrhizae	6 g

All the above drugs are to be decocted in water for oral administration.

Chinese Patent Medicine

1) *Zangqingguo chongji*. A block is dissolved in boiled water and is taken three times daily.

2) Recipe:

Fructus Arctii	9 g
Periostracum Cicadae	4.5 g
Radix Glycyrrhizae	6 g

All the above drugs are to be decocted in water for oral administration.

2) **invasion of the larynx by wind - heat**

Main Symptoms and Signs: Hoarseness or pain in articulation may occur. Dryness and a sensation of burning heat as well as sore throat may be present. Swelling of, or yellow - white pus specks on the laryngeal mucous membrane with exudates attached may be seen. There are accompanying symptoms such as fever, cough, yellow sputum or dyspnea. The tongue is red with yellow fur on it and the pulse is floating and rapid.

Therapeutic Principles: Disperse pathogenic wind and heat and remove toxic substances to promote subsidence of swelling.

Recipe: *Powder of lonicera and forsythia*

Flos Lonicerae	24 g
Fructus Forsythiae	15 g
Rhizoma Phragmitis	15 g
Fructus Arctii	9 g
Herba Schizonepetae	9 g
Semen Sojae Praeparatum	9 g
Herba Menthae	9 g
Radix Platycodi	9 g

Herba Lophatheri	9 g
Radix Glycyrrhizae	6 g

All the above drugs are to be decocted in water for oral administration.

Modification: For those with excessive heat, add 30 grams of *Gypsum Fibrosum*, 15 g of *Cortex Moutan Radicis*. For pain in speaking, and reddish swelling in the arytenoid area, add 15 g of *Radix Scrophulariae*, 30 g of *Radix Isatidis*, 18 g of *Herba Violae*. For mucous cough with yellowish phlegm, add 9 g of *Bulbus Fritillariae Thunbergii*, 18 g of *Fructus Trichosanthis*. For dry stool, add 9 g of *Radix et Rhizoma Rhei* and 9 g of *Mirabilitum*.

Chinese Patent Medicine

Niuhuang jie du pian. Take 6 tablets or one bolus with warm water, twice daily.

Jin sang kui yin wan. Take one bolus each tim, twice a day.

3) Recipe:

Herba Taraxaci	15 g
Herba Andrographitis	15 g
Flos Chrysanthemi	15 g
Radix Isatidis	15 g
Fructus Arctiiariae	15 g
Radix Scrophulariae	15 g

All the above drugs are to be decocted in water for oral administration.

2. External Treatment

1) **herbal steam inhalation**

Recipe:

Herba Menthae	9 g
Herba Agastachis seu Pogostemonis	9 g
Herba Eupatorii	9 g
Flos Chrysanthemi	15 g
Flos Lonicerae	15 g

All the above drugs are to be decocted in water to make 200 ml of decoction and, after being filtered, it is used for steam inhalation or ultrasonic spray inhalation. The decoction is used as three separate doses.

2) **insufflation of powder drug**

Blow *Bing peng san* into the larynx several times daily.

Acupuncture and Moxibustion

1) Shallow puncture with blood out: Refer to *Acute Epiglottis* for the performance.

2) Acupuncture: Select the points **Hégǔ(LI4)**, **Rényíng(ST9)**, **Shuǐtū(ST10)**, **Chǐzé(LU5)**, **Tiāntū(RN22)** and use two to three of them each time with reducing technique, once a day.

Chapter Eleven
Acute Subglottic Laryngitis

Acute subglottic laryngitis refers to the acute inflammation of the mucous membrane below the glottis with the main symptoms of fever, hoarse voice, dyspnea due to retention of sputum, and even difficult breathing. It usually occurs in infants younger than 3 years old with the characteristics of sudden onset and fast course of the disease. In traditional Chinese medicine, it belongs to the category of "jí hóu fēng" (sudden obstruction of the throat).

ETIOLOGY AND PATHOGENESIS

The five solid organs and six hollow organs of the infants are still near their beginning in *yin* and *yang* for they are just formed but not perfect, or perfect but not strong. Their ability is too weak to endure cold or heat in the outer environment. In case of invasion by wind – heat evils, their reaction is usually very acute. With accumulation of sputum and heat below the glottis the disease occurs.

MAIN SYMPTOMS AND SIGNS

1. Sudden, continuous fever, hoarse voice, coughing like a dog's barking, dyspnea due to rhonchus.
2. Breathing in difficulty, in a severe case, with the sign of triconcave for suction of the air.
3. Examination of the throat shows congestion and swelling of the vocal cords, and more serious below glottis.
4. Possibly accompanied by irritability, cold sweat all over, pale complexion and lips, and indistinct pulse.

Chapter Eleven

DIFFERENTIATION AND TREATMENT OF COMMON SYNDROMES

1. Internal Treatment

Therapeutic Principles: Clarify heat and resolve toxins, and reduce phlegm for resuscitation.

Recipe: *Qing wen bai du san*

Cornu Rhinocerotis	1 g
Cortex Moutan Radicis	6 g
Radix Paeoniae Rubra	6 g
Rhizoma Coptidis	6 g
Radix Scutellariae	6 g
Rhizoma Anemarrhenae	6 g
Fructus Gardeniae	9 g
Fructus Forsythiae	9 g
Radix Glycyrrhizae	15 g
Radix Scrophulariae	6 g
Periostracum Cicadae	6 g

All the above drugs are to be decocted in water for oral administration.

Modification: For excessiveness of sputum and secretion, add 6 g of *Concretio Siliceae Bambusae* and 6 g of *Bulbus Fritillariae Thunbergii*. For rapid respiration, grind the tablets of *An gong niuhuang wan* into powder and mix it in boiled water for pouring down the throats of children patients the dose is varied according to the age of children and severity of their symptoms), and have the surgical operation o tracheotomy if need arises.

Chinese Patent Medicine

Liu shen wan. Take either as many pills as the number of years of the age or 3 – 5 pills with boiled water.

2. External Treatment

Pay close attention to the course of the disease and get ready for a surgical operation if necessary.

Acupuncture and Moxibustion

1) Shallow puncture with blood out: Refer to *Acute Epiglottitis*.
2) Acupuncture: Select **Hégǔ**(**LI**4), **Shàoshāng**(**LU**11), **Shàozé**(**SI**1), **Qūchí**(**LI**11) and **Fēnglóng**(**ST**40) and use two to three of them each time with he method of purgation, twice a day.

Chapter Twelve
Chronic Laryngitis

Chronic laryngitis, a chronic inflammation of the laryngeal mucous membrane, can involve submucous layer and intralaryngeal muscles. Low voice, hoarseness and long duration are is main clinical manifestations. It falls into the category of "jīu yīn" (long–time loss of voice) in traditional Chinese medicine.

ETIOLOGY AND PATHOGENESIS

The Throat is nourished by *yin* essence of the lung and kidney. With insufficiency of *yin* essence, the throat fails to be nourished. *Yin* deficiency results in internal heat, causing asthenic ire to flare up to the throat and the remaining evils to stagnate there. In this way the disease occurs.

MAIN SYMPTOMS AND SIGNS

1. The voice is neither loud nor clear but hoarse and tough, or very low.
2. Dryness and itching in the larynx with wheezing sound, or feeling of a foreign body there.
3. The vocal cords are congested, dark–red or reddish, or with expansion of the cabolusary of mucous membrane. The secretion in the glottis looks wire-drawn. Both the ventricular bands and arytenoid area look dark–reddish due to congestion. The glottis can not be closed completely with a fine fissure between two sides.
4. Little moisture on pharyngeal mucous membrane for lack of essence of secretion as well as diffuse congestion of it.
5. Accompanied by thirsty, drinking little water, feverish sensation in the palm and sole, dry coughing with little sputum, reddish and tender tongue with thin, whitish fur, thin and rapid pulse.

MAIN POINTS OF DIAGNOSIS

1. This disease is mostly seen in the professionals who make overuse or misuse of their voice.
2. The patient's voice is soft but husky and of low pitch. He or she cannot talk for a long time or has aphonia in a severe case.
3. The patient has dark redness and swelling in the vocal cords and aryepiglottic folds or the ventricular bands. The vocal cords are thickened or with noduli and polyps on them. The glottides cannot be completely closed.
4. The patient feels itching and uncomfortable or has a sensation of foreign body in the throat.

DIFFERENTIATION AND TREATMENT OF COMMON SYNDROMES

1. Internal Treatment

1) yin deficiency of both the lung and kidney

Main Symptoms and Signs: The voice remains hoarse for a long time and cannot be raised. The vocal cords are congested and become light red with thickened rims. The patient feels itching and has a sensation of burning heat and slight pain in the throat. The accompanying symptoms are cough with little sputum but tidal fever in the afternoon. The tongue is red and the pulse taut and thready.

Therapeutic Principles: Nourish the lung and kidney and relieve sore throat to restore voice.

Recipe: *Lily bulb decoction for strengthening the lung*

Bulbus Lillii	15 g
Radix Rehmanniae	15 g
Radix Ophiopogonis	15 g
Radix Scrophulariae	15 g
Radix Angelicae Sinensis	15 g
Radix Paeoniae Alba	15 g
Bulbus Fritillariae Cirrhosae	9 g

Radix Platycodi	6 g
Radix Glycyrrhizae	6 g
Radix Rehmanniae Praeparata	18 g

All the above drugs are to be decocted in water for oral administration.

Modification: For those with lassitude of the loins and legs, and burning sensation of the palms and soles, add 9 g of *Fructus Lycii*, 30 g of *Fructus Mori*, 9 g of *Cortex Phellodendri*. For those with feeling of short breath and fatigued and dry cough with little sputum, add 9 g of *Radix Ginseng* and 30 g of *Rhizoma Dioscoreae*.

Chinese Patent Medicine

Jin sang qing yin wan. Take one bolus, twice a day.

Tie di wan. Take 2 boluses, 3 times a day.

Yang yin qing fei wan. Take 2 boluses, twice a day.

2) **qi deficiency of both the lung and spleen**

Main Symptoms and Signs: The patient has a hoarse voice for a long time and the hoarseness is aggravated by overwork. His speech cannot last long and his voice is low. Congestion of the laryngeal mucous membrane is present. The vocal cords are relaxed or have hydrops along the edges. The glottides cannot be closed completely. The tongue is reddish with indentations, along its edges, the fur is thin and white. Thready and feeble pulse.

Therapeutic Principles: Reinforce middle − *jiao* and replenish *qi* and strengthen the throat to improve voice.

Recipe: *Decoction for reinforcing middle − jiao and replenishing qi with additional ingredients*

Radix Astragali seu Hedysari	24 g
Radix Glycyrrhizae Praeparata	9 g
Radix Ginseng	9 g
Pericarpium Citri Reticulatae	9 g
Rhizoma Cimicifugae	9 g
Radix Bupleuri	9 g
Rhizoma Atractylodis Macrocephalae	9 g
Fructus Chebulae	9 g
Rhizoma Acori Graminei	9 g
Radix Angelicae Sinensis	15 g

All the above drugs are to be decocted in water for oral administration.

3) **stagnation of qi and stasis of blood**

Main Symptoms and Signs: The voice remains hoarse for a long time. The vocal cords become thickened, dark-red and congested, with polypoid changes and polyps along its edges and the ventricular bands thickened, the mucous membrane of the arytenoid region congested. The tongue is red or dark-red and the pulse taut and thready.

Therapeutic Principles: Promote *blood* circulation and remove *blood* stasis to restore voice.

Recipe: *Decoction for removing blood stasis in the epiglottis*

Radix Angelicae Sinensis	15 g
Radix Paeoniae Rubra	15 g
Radix Scrophulariae	15 g
Semen Persicae	9 g
Flos Carthami	9 g
Radix Platycodi	9 g
Radix Rehmanniae	9 g
Radix Bupleuri	9 g
Fructus Aurantii	12 g
Radix Glycyrrhizae	6 g

All the above drugs are to be decocted in water for oral administration.

Modification: For those with hoarseness for a long time, add 9 grams of *Periostracum Cicadae*, 9 grams of *Semen Sterculiae Scaphigerae* and 9 grams of *Semen Oroxyli*. For those with severe hydrops of the vocal cords, add 30 grams of *Semen Coicis* and 15 grams of *Rhizoma Alismatis*. For those with nodules and polyps on the vocal cords, add 15 grams of *Os Costaziae*, 9 grams of *Bombyx Batryticatus*, 9 grams of *Herba Lycopodii* and 9 grams of *Rhizoma Sparganii*. For those with intense fire due to *yin* deficiency, add 9 grams of *Cortex Moutan Radicis*, 9 grams of *Rhizoma Anemarrhenae* and 9 grams of *Cortex Phellodendri*.

2. External Treatment

1) *Baimao xiakucao* or *Yin huang ye*

Spray 10 ml with ultrasonic waves and insufflate it in the throat, twice a day.

2) Mix the powder of all the following with honey to make pellets weighing 6 g each:

Radix Adenophorae Strictae	45 g
Radix Platycodi	45 g
Fructus Chebulae	60 g
Borax	7.5 g

Keep one pellet in the mouth and then swallow slowly after it is dissolved twice a day.

Acupuncture and Moxibustion

1) Acupuncture: Select the points **Rényíng(ST9)**, **Tiāntū(RN22)**, **Shuǐtū(ST10)**, **Lièquē(LU7)**, and **Hégǔ(LI4)** and use two to three of them each time, retaining the needle for 20 minutes, once a day.

2) Moxibustion: Select **Tiāntū(RN22)**, **Qìshè(ST11)**, and **Xuánjī(RN21)**, and use them for moxibustion with moxa cones. Cover the points with slices of ginger before treatment.

Chapter Thirteen
Chronic Hypertrophic Laryngitis

Chronic hypertrophic laryngitis refers to hyperplastic pathologic change of the laryngeal mucous membrane, clinically manifested by prolonged hoarseness, guttural dryness and a sensation of a foreign body in the throat due to general weakness and stagnation of pathogenic evils for prolonged illness. In traditional Chinese medicine it belongs to the category of "Màn hóu yīn" (chronic aphonia due to throat disease).

ETIOLOGY AND PATHOGENESIS

It occurs due to repeated attacks of acute laryngitis, or deficiency in the lung, spleen and kidney for prolonged illness with stagnant evil factors, or due to disharmony of *qi* and *blood* resulting in stagnation of *qi* and *blood* and accumulation of sputum in the throat.

MAIN SYMPTOMS AND SIGNS

1. Prolonged hoarseness, which aggravates when one speaks a little more.
2. Sputum adheres to the throat and is hard to cough up. The throat feels dry, and there is a sensation of a foreign body in it.
3. The laryngeal mucous membrane is hyperplastic, dark – reddish and deficient in moisture. The vocal cords show hyperplastic change. The ventricular bands look exceeding. The mucous membrane between arytenoid parts look hyperplastic and dark – reddish as well. The glottis can not be closed and with viscous sputum attached.

4. Dark – reddish tongue with thin, whitish fur, and sunken and thin pulse.

5. Accompanied by pale complexion, general weakness, poor appetite, abdominal distention, insomnia and dreaminess.

DIFFERENTIATION AND TREATMENT OF COMMON SYNDROMES

1. Internal Treatment

Therapeutic Principles: Activate *blood* and eliminate *blood* stasis; expel sputum and ease up the voice.

Recipe: *Huiyan zhuyu tang*

Radix Angelicae Sinensis	15 g
Radix Paeoniae Rubra	15 g
Semen Persicae	9 g
Flos Carthami	9 g
Radix Scrophulariae	15 g
Fructus Aurantii	15 g
Radix Bupleuri	9 g
Radix Rehmanniae	15 g
Radix Glycyrrhizae	6 g
Periostracum Cicadae	4.5 g
Bombyx Batryticatus	15 g

All the above drugs are to be decocted in water for oral administration.

Modification: For much dryness of the throat, add 15 g of *Bulbus Lillii* and 9 g of *Fructus Canarii*. For hypertrophic mucous membrane, add 9 g of *Spina Gleditsiae* and 30 g of *Os Costaziae*. For flatulence, add 9 g of *Rhizoma Atractylodis Macrocephalae* and 30 g of *Semen Coicis*. For abundant expectoration, add 18 g of *Fructus Trichosanthis* and 12 g of *Radix Peucedani*.

Chinese Patent Medicine

Jin sang san jie wan. One bolus, twice a day.

Tie di wan. Same as that in *Chronic Laryngitis*.

2. External Treatment

1) **insufflation**: Refer to *Chronic Laryngitis*.

2) **paste**: Put *Qing fei gao* on the chest, once a day. Or put *Na qi gao* below umbilicus, once a day.

Acupuncture and Moxibustion

Refer to *Chronic Laryngitis*.

Chapter Fourteen
Atrophic Laryngitis

Atrophic laryngitis is a chronic, progressive, atrophic pathologic change occurring in the soft tissue of the throat. Clinically it is characterized by dryness, discomfort, burning pain and hoarseness in the throat. It belongs to the category of "Màn hóu yīn" (chronic laryngoaphasia) and "Wěi zhèng" (flaccidity syndrome) in traditional Chinese medicine.

ETIOLOGY AND PATHOGENESIS

It is related to protracted illness with no proper treatment, or general weakness, or pollution of the environment, or the attack of the exogenous evil of dryness, or radiation damage resulting in insufficiency of *yin* – essence, accumulation of endogenous and exogenous dryness – evils in the throat, myolemma burned by asthenic fire, unprosperousness of *qi* and *blood* and tissue atrophy.

MAIN SYMPTOMS AND SIGNS

1. A tickling sensation in the throat, dry cough or spasmodic cough with a little mucous sputum, or coughing out crust mixed with streaks of blood at the rising hour in the morning.
2. A dry or hoarse voice, or even loss of voice; voice improves temporarily if pieces of crust are coughed out; speaking with difficulty or a painful sensation.
3. Laryngeal mucosa is dry, deep red in color, rough or shining, thin or atrophic, often accompanied with yellow or green crust, shrinkage of the vocal cord and dysphasia of the glottis.

4. It is often observed that mucosa on the back wall of the pharynx and in the nasal cavity is dry or less moist, or atrophic with pieces of crust.

DIFFERENTIATION AND TREATMENT OF COMMON SYNDROMES

1. Internal Treatment

1) the lung-dryness syndrome due to *yin* deficiency

Main Symptoms and Signs: A dry and tickling sensation in the throat, cough productive of a small amount of mucous sputum, a dry voice which is hoarse sometimes, speaking with a dry painful sensation, dry laryngeal mucosa, thinned vocal cord with weak tension, crust in the cricoarytenoid area, nose dryness and discomfort, shortness of breath, lassitude, red and delicate tongue with little dy fur, thready and rapid pulse.

Therapeutic Principles: Nourish *yin* to moisten the lung, and remove dryness to restore the sound.

Recipe: *Yang yin qing fei tang*

Radix Scrophulariae	15 g
Radix Rehmanniae	15 g
Radix Ophiopogonis	15 g
Cortex Moutan Radicis	15 g
Bulbus Fritillariae	15 g
Herba Menthae	9 g
Radix Glycyrrhizae	9 g
Radix Scutellariae	9 g
Cortex Mori Radicis	15 g
Radix Adenophorae Strictae	30 g

All the above drugs are to be decocted in water for oral administration.

Modification: For dryness with much crust, add *Fructus Ligustri Lucidi* 30 g and *Colla Corii Asini* 15 g. For productive cough with blood streaks, add *Rhizoma Imperatae* 30 g and *Pollen Typhae* 9 g.

Chinese Patent Medicine

Qin hua wan. Take one bolus each time, have it melt slowly in the mouth before swallowing, several times a day.

Liuwei dihuang wan. Take one bolus each time, three times a day.

2) **weakness of both the lung and kidney**

Main Symptoms and Signs: Cough due to a tickling sensation in the throat or spasmodic cough which is relieved after coughing up pieces of crust, blood-streaked sputum with crust, hoarseness or aphonia, shining atrophic mucosa with yellow and green crust sticking on, thin shrinking vocal cord, mucous atrophy on the back wall of the pharynx and in the nasal cavity, lumbago and lassitude, feverish sensation in the palms and soles, red tongue with little fur, taut and thready pulse.

Therapeutic Principles: Nourish the lung and the kidney; moisten the throat to restore the sound.

Recipe: *Baihe gu jin tang*

Bulbus Lillii	24 g
Radix Rehmanniae Praeparata	18 g
Radix Rehmanniae	15 g
Radix Ophiopogonis	15 g
Radix Angelicae Sinensis	15 g
Radix Paeoniae Alba	15 g
Bulbus Fritillariae	9 g
Radix Scrophulariae	15 g
Radix Pseudostellariae	24 g
Radix Glycyrrhizae Praeparata	9 g

All the above drugs are to be decocted in water for oral administration.

Modification: For severe atrophic mucosa, add *Semen Cuscutae* 30 g and *Fructus Mori*. For poor appetite, add *Fructus Crataegi* 15 g and *Rhizoma Dioscoreae* 30 g. For blood-streaked sputum, add *Radix Rubiae* 9 g and *Herba Agrimoniae* 30 g.

Chinese Patent Medicine

Refer to that in Chapter thirteen.

2. **External Treatment**

1) **aerosol inhalation**: Decoct 30 g of *Herba Cistanchis*, 30 g of *Bulbus Lillii*

and 15 g of *Herba Menthae* into 100 – 150 ml of liquor, to inhale by ultrasonic nebulization once or twice a day, 20 ml each time.

2) **perlingual therapy**: Hold *Shishuang pian* in the mouth several times a day.

Acupuncture and Moxibustion

It is advisable to choose 2 to 3 points each time among **Tiāntū(RN22)**, **Hégǔ(LI4)**, **Liánquán(RN23)**, **Tàiyuān(LU9)**, **Fèishū(BL13)**, **Píshū(BL20)** and **Zúsānlǐ(ST36)**. Puncture with reinforcing technique once a day.

Chapter Fifteen
Rhythmic Palatopharyngolaryngeal Muscular Clonus

The chief manifestations of this disease are fine rhythmic clonic contractions of muscles of soft palate, uvula, pharynx or larynx, and involuntary phonation of croup sound. The affected part is chiefly at the brain stem, especially the inferior olivary body. The pathogenesis of this disease is at present not well known. There is no such corresponding term in traditional Chinese medicine. From theoretical point of view, larynx has the distributions of lung, liver and kidney meridians and collaterals and this disease is treated accordingly.

ETIOLOGY AND PATHOGENESIS

The insufficiency of he liver and kidney; the failure of dispersion of pulmonary *qi*; the loss of wetness of pharynx and larynx; the clonic spasm of muscles.

DIFFERENTIATION AND TREATMENT OF COMMON SYNDROMES

1) **the deficiency of kidney *yin*, and the internal agitation of hepatic wind**

The deficiency of kidney *yin*, the kidney fluid can not nourish the liver, the irritant flow of endogenous hepatic wind, the liver *fire* injures the lung, the failure of dispersion of lung *qi*, and the loss of wetness of pharynx and larynx.

Main Symptoms and Signs: Sound like "Ge – Ge" produced in larynx, slurred speech, tremble of Adam's apple, the "Ge – Ge" sound alleviated during talking, feeding or sound sleep, dryness of mouth and pharynx, vexation and hotness over palms, soles and the heart, insomnia and dreaminess, muscular twitching, trembling of hands or feet. Aching and flaccidity of loin and knee. Red tongue proper with little fur, taut and thready pulse.

Therapeutic Principles: Nourish the kidney and liver essence, to moist the lung and extinguish the wind.

Recipe: *Yang yin qing fei tang*

Radix Rehmanniae	24 g
Radix Ophiopogonis	24 g
Radix Platycodi	6 g
Radix Glycyrrhizae	3 g
Scorpio (powder)	6 g
Centipedium (powder)	4 g

The first four drugs are to be decocted in water and the other two ground into powder. Mix the powder into the decoction for oral administration.

Modification: For prominent vexation and insomnia, add *Fructus Jujubae Indici* and *Fructus Gardeniae*; for conspicuous muscular twitching or trembling of hands and feet, add *Concha Ostreae*, *Os Draconis*, *earthworm*; for obvious dryness of mouth and pharynx vexation and anger tendency, add *Radix Bupleuri*, *Semen Oroxyli*, *Rhizoma Anemarrhenae*, *Fructus Gardeniae*; for constipation, add *Radix et Rhizoma Rhei* and *Rhizoma Anemarrhenae*.

Chinese Patent Medicine

Liuwei dihuang wan. One bolus, t.i.d., *Scorpion and centipede powder* 2 g each.

Acupuncture and Moxibustion

Shènshū(BL23), **Gānshū**(BL18), **Tàixī**(KI3) are needled with reinforcing method; **Tàichōng**(LR3), **Xíngjiān**(LR2), **Tiāntū**(RN22), and **Liánquán**(RN23) punctured with reducing method.

2) **insufficiency of kidney** *yang*, **with upward disturbance of wind and phlegm**

Etiology And Pathogenesis: The insufficiency of kidney *yang*, the failure of transference of fluid which accumulated and resulted phlegm. The up-surge of wind-phlegm; the dysfunction of lung in cleansing and descending the qi, and thus with the pharynx and larynx affected.

Main Symptoms and Signs: Thyroid cartilage clonus, production of "Ge – Ge" sound, continuous and persistent, temporary remissions while eating or drinking or during sleep, spitting of saliva or sputum, oppressive sensation in the chest, chilliness over the waist and back, muscular twitching, urination clear and not short, stool soft; The condition exacerbates after exposure to cold. Plump with teeth indentations over the margin o tongue proper, white and moist tongue coating, deep and relaxed pulse.

Therapeutic Principles: Warm up the kidney and assist the *yang*; resolve the phlegm and extinguish the wind.

Recipe: *Zhen wu tang* et *Er chen tang* with modification

Radix Aconiti Praeparata	12 g
Rhizoma Atractylodis Macrocephalae	15 g
Poria	24 g
Pericarpium Citri Reticulatae	12 g
Rhizoma Pinelliae	12 g
Bulbus Fritillariae Thunbergii	10 g
Bulbus Lillii	30 g
Bombyx Batryticatus	12 g
Earthworm	12 g
Concha Ostreae	24 g

All the above drugs are to be decocted in water for oral administration.

Modification: For clonus of thyroid cartilage with prominent "Ge – Ge" sound, add *scorpion and centipede powder*; for aversion to cold, pronounced loose stool, add *Rhizoma Zingiberis Recens*; for excessive salivation and sputum, add *Fructus Evodiae* and *Cardamon seed*.

Chinese Patent Medicine

Jin gui shen qi wan. One bolus t.i.d. Powder of *earthworm*, *centipede*, *scorpion* 3 g each, three times a day.

Acupuncture and Moxibustion

Guānyuán(RN4), **Mìngmén**(DU4), and **Zúsānlǐ**(ST36) applied with moxibustion; **Zhōngwǎn**(RN12), **Fēnglóng**(ST40), **Tiāntū**(RN22), and **Liánquán**(RN23) punctured with reducing method.

Chapter Sixteen
Polyp of the Vocal Cord

Polyp of the vocal cord refers to the grey or reddish vegetation with pedunculus on the vocal cords, which takes place often on the section of the edge of one vocal cord between its midpoint and the position one third distance away from the joint of the vocal cods due to improper sound producing method or overuse of the voice, lack of treatment for chronic aphonia, or loss and deficiency in the viscera, with the main symptoms of hoarse voice and difficulty in speaking. In traditional Chinese medicine it belongs to the category of "Màn hóu yīn" (chronic aphonia due to throat disease) and "Shēng sī".

ETIOLOGY AND PATHOGENESIS

It is due to deficiency of the lung and spleen, or external invasion by wind-evils, or injury to the throat by singing, or injury to *qi* by speaking too much or making sound too hard, *qi* and *blood* become disharmonious, and dispersion of water and dampness becomes out of order, resulting in stagnation of *qi* and *blood* as well as accumulation of water and dampness in the passage of throat, which eventually forms the polyp there.

MAIN POINTS OF DIAGNOSIS

1. Intermittent huskiness or hoarseness, difficulty in speaking o a feeling of suffocation, or even losing voice.
2. Coughing due to a tickling sensation, a feeling of a foreign body or an obstruction in the throat.

3. Congestion and dark — redness of the vocal cords, or swelling of the mucous membrane, or normal color of the vocal cords.

4. Polyp with pedunculus, white or red, or pale and with the boundary fish — belly alike, is situated on the section of the edge of one vocal cod between the midpoint and the position one third distance from the joint o the vocal cords.

5. Usually, polyp of the vocal cod occurs in the middle — aged or the young; red polyp often occurs in the female.

DIFFERENTIATION AND TREATMENT OF COMMON SYNDROMES

1. Internal Treatment

1) deficiency of the lung and spleen

Main Symptoms and Signs: Difficult speaking with a low and hoarse voice, polyp shaped as a bubble or fish — belly, inability to have a long dialogue, feeling fatigued, loss of appetite, light reddish tongue with thin, whitish fur, thin and weak pulse.

Therapeutic Principles: Strengthen the spleen and nourish *qi* ; promote diuresis and disperse the accumulation of evils.

Recipe: *Si jun zi tang* et *Si ling san*, modified.

Radix Ginseng	9 g
Rhizoma Atractylodis Macrocephalae	9 g
Poria	15 g
Rhizoma Alismatis	15 g
Polyporus Umbellatus	9 g
Semen Sterculiae Scaphigerae	9 g
Periostracum Cicadae	4.5 g
Semen Coicis	30 g
Radix Scrophulariae	15 g
Radix Glycyrrhizae	6 g

All the above drugs are to be decocted in water for oral administration.

Modification: For loss of appetite and loose stool, add 30 g of *Rhizoma Dioscoreae*, 9 g of *Radix Aucklandiae* and 9 g of *Pericarpium Citri Reticu-*

latae. For congestion of vocal cords and expansion of cabolusary, add 9 g of *Herba Lycopi* and 15 g of *Radix Paeoniae Rubra*. For solid polyp, add 9 g of *Spina Gleditsiae* and 9 g of *Bombyx Batryticatus*.

2) **stagnation of *qi* and *blood***

Main Symptoms and Signs: Chronic raucitas or dim timbre, violet reddish or light reddish polyp, reddish tongue with petechiae and little fur, and sunken and thin pulse.

Therapeutic Principles: Activate *blood* and eliminate the stagnation; disperse the accumulation of evils and easing up the voice.

Recipe: *Huiyan zhu yu tang*

Radix Angelicae Sinensis	15 g
Radix Paeoniae Rubra	15 g
Semen Persicae	9 g
Flos Carthami	6 g
Radix Bupleuri	9 g
Fructus Aurantii	12 g
Radix Scrophulariae	15 g
Radix Rehmanniae	12 g
Radix Platycodi	6 g
Herba Lycopi	9 g
Rhizoma Ligustici Chuanxiong	9 g
Bombyx Batryticatus	9 g

All the above drugs are to be decocted in water for oral administration.

Modification: For polyp with much redness and swelling, add 9 g of *Radix Scutellariae* and 24 g of *Flos Lonicerae*. For feeling fatigued and shortness of breath, add 9 g of *Radix Ginseng* and 15 g of *Rhizoma Polygonati*. For feeling dry in the throat, add 18 g of *Fructus Ligustri Lucidi* and 15 g of *Herba Dendrobii*.

Chinese Patent Medicine

Qing yin wan. Take one bolus each time, twice a day.

Jin san san ji wan. Take one bolus each time, three times a day.

2. External Treatment

A surgical operation is needed to take off the polyp when the course of the disease is longer than 2 months.

Acupuncture and Moxibustion

Select the points **Rényíng (ST9)**, **Shuǐtū (ST10)**, **Liánquán (RN23)**, **Tiāntū (RN22)**, and **Fēnglóng(ST40)** and use 3 of them each time with the method of purgation, once a day.

Chapter Seventeen
Vocal Nodules

Vocal nodules, also called nodules of the singer, refer to the grain – shaped, usually symmetrical overshoots on the epithelium of the bilateral vocal cords's edges. Those nodules often occur in actors and actresses, teachers, salesmen and other professionals who work using their sound frequently. In traditional Chinese medicine, it belongs to the category of "Màn hóu yīn" (chronic aphonia due to laryngitis) and "Jiu yīn" (prolonged aphonia).

ETIOLOGY AND PATHOGENESIS

The condition result from disharmony of *qi* and *blood*, uneven flow in channels and collaterals, and obstruction of the throat by turbid sputum due to overuse of the voice, or crying too loudly, or consumptive diseases in the viscera, or injury of *qi* and *blood* due to improper method of producing sound.

MAIN SYMPTOMS AND SIGNS

1. The voice is not loud and clear, or "broken" on making a loud voice, or very hoarse with sputum attached. It becomes normal temporarily after clearing the throat by giving a slight cough.
2. The segment of edge of the vocal cord from the midpoint to where one third distance from the joint is not smooth. There appear symmetric, pinpoint – shaped overshoots, which are red or white, hard or attached with viscous fluid.
3. There are two chinks in the glottis in front of and behind the nodules.

4. Through an dynamic laryngoscopy, synchronized oscillations of the vocal cord are seen but waves of mucous membrane disappear near the nodules.

5. Uneasiness in the throat and inability to rid the sputum by coughing.

6. Feeling fatigued and short of breath, light reddish tongue with thin, whitish fur, and thin pulse.

DIFFERENTIATION AND TREATMENT OF COMMON SYNDROMES

1. Internal Treatment

Therapeutic Principles: Harmonize *qi* and *blood*, expel sputum and disperse the accumulation of evils.

Recipe: *Si jun zi tang*

Radix Ginseng	9 g
Rhizoma Atractylodis Macrocephalae	9 g
Poria	15 g
Radix Angelicae Sinensis	15 g
Rhizoma Ligustici Chuanxiong	9 g
Radix Paeoniae Rubra	15 g
Semen Persicae	9 g
Flos Carthami	4.5 g
Periostracum Cicadae	4.5 g
Radix Rehmanniae	15 g
Bombyx Batryticatus	9 g
Os Costaziae	30 g

All the above drugs are to be decocted in water for oral administration.

Modification: For edema due to dampness, add *Rhizoma Atractylodis* 9 g and *Rhizoma Dioscoreae* 30 g. For hyperplastic vocal cords, add 15 g of *Spica Prunellae* and 30 g of *Thallus Laminariae seu Eckloniae* 30 g. For solid nodules, add *Spina Gleditsiae* 9 g and *Sargassum* 30 g.

2. External Treatment

It is preferable to perform a laryngomicrosurgical operation. Refer to **Chapter Sixteen**.

Acupuncture and Moxibustion

The points are **Rényíng(ST9)**, **Fútū(LI18)**, **Píshū(BL20)**, **Shuǐtū(ST10)**, **Hégǔ (LI4)**, **Zúsānlǐ(ST36)**, **Fēnglóng(ST40)** and **Zhàohǎi(KI6)**. 3 to 4 points are selected each time. The treatment is given once every day with the needles retained for 30 minutes.

Chapter Eighteen
Vocal Edema

Vocal edema refers to water accumulation of mucous subepithelial Ranke's layer of the vocal cord. Clinically it is characterized by hoarseness, marginal edema of the vocal cord and glottidodysraphism. It belongs to the category of "Màn hóu yīn" and "Shŭi zhŏng" in traditional Chinese medicine.

ETIOLOGY AND PATHOGENESIS

It is due to dysfunction of the lung, spleen and kidney, and disorder of transportation and distribution of body fluid; or de to improper use of voice, excessive use of voice and impairment of the vocal cod, which result in incoordination between *qi* and *blood*, rough flow of channels and vessels, and accumulation of fluid in the throat.

MAIN SYMPTOMS AND SIGNS

1. Hoarseness, no improvement with the time passing by, usually seen in cases of excessive use of voice.
2. Local or whole-length edema process on one side or both sides of the vocal cord, pale color, semitransparent, even floating with airflow in breathing.
3. Often accompanied with lassitude, cold sensation in the limbs, anorexia and loose bowel.
4. Slight red and enlarged tongue, thin and white tongue coating, slippery or deep thready pulse.

Vocal Edema

DIFFERENTIATION AND TREATMENT OF COMMON SYNDROMES

1. Internal Treatment

Therapeutic Principles: Strengthen the spleen and replenish he kidney, and induce diuresis to alleviate edema.

Recipe: *Si jun zi tang* et *Zhen wu tang*, modified.

Radix Ginseng	9 g
Rhizoma Atractylodis Macrocephalae	9 g
Poria	15 g
Radix Aconiti Praeparata	9 g
Radix Paeoniae Alba	15 g
Rhizoma Zingiberis Recens	9 g
Ramulus Cinnamomi	9 g
Herba Epimedii	9 g
Semen Coicis	30 g

All the above drugs are to be decocted in water for oral administration.

Modification: For general weakness, add 18 g of *Radix Astragali seu Hedysari*. For congestion of throat, add 9 g of *Radix Scutellariae* and 9 g of *Cortex Phellodendri*. For anorexia and loose stool, add 15 g of *Semen Dolichoris Macrocephalae* and 15 g of *Rhizoma Alismatis*.

Chinese Patent Medicine

Ji sheng shen qi wan. Take one bolus each time, twice a day.

2. External Treatment

1) *Baimao xiakucao* or *Yin huang ye*. Spray 10 ml with ultrasonic waves and insufflate it in the throat, twice a day.

2) Mix the powder o all the following with honey to make pellets weighing 6 g each.

Radix Adenophorae Strictae	45 g
Radix Platycodi	45 g
Fructus Chebulae	60 g

Borax   7.5 g

Keep the pellet in the mouth and then swallow slowly after it is dissolved, twice a day.

Acupuncture and Moxibustion

1) Select **Rénying(ST9)**, **Tiāntū(RN22)**, **Shuǐtū(ST10)**, **Lièquē(LU7)**, and **Hégǔ(LI4)** and use 2 – 3 of them each time, retaining the needles for 20 minutes, once a day.

2) Select **Tiāntū(RN22)**, **Qìshè(ST11)**, and **Xuánjī(RN21)**, and apply moxa cones on points, with ginger slices covered on them. 7 cones ignited for each point, once a day.

Chapter Nineteen
Vocal Mucosal Hemorrhage

Vocal mucosal hemorrhage is not uncommon in the clinic, it is characterized by huskiness, difficulty in vocalization or sore throat on sudden exertion of vocal cord. Before the onset it is often accompanied with upper respiratory tract infection and menstrual period. It belongs to some cases of "Bào yīn" (sudden loss of voice) in traditional Chinese medicine.

ETIOLOGY AND PATHOGENESIS

It is related to insufficiency of both the spleen and the kidney, insufficiency of essence and blood due to the kidney deficiency and dysfunction of *blood* absorption due to insufficiency of the kidney, causing hemorrhage of the vessels when one suddenly sings, shouts, coughs and sneezes with the blood vessels impaired.

MAIN SYMPTOMS AND SIGNS

1. Huskiness or difficulty in vocalization, especially in sudden forceful sound production, pain in the throat area, difficulty in speaking.
2. There are irregular bright red or purplish red spots on one side or both sides of the vocal cord, higher than the surface of the vocal cord, with clear margins; the color may become dark red or brown black when the duration is long.
3. Accompanied with dim complexion, shortness of breath and weakness, pain in the loins and knees, and anorexia.

4. Often elated to recent infection of the upper respiratory tract or coming menstruation.

5. Light red tongue or with petechiae on it, thin – white tongue coating, deep thready pulse.

DIFFERENTIATION AND TREATMENT OF COMMON SYNDROMES

1. Internal Treatment

Therapeutic Principles: Remove heat from the *blood* to stop bleeding, and remove the *blood* stasis to restore the sound.

Recipe:

Radix Rehmanniae	15 g
Cortex Moutan Radicis	15 g
Radix Paeoniae Alba	15 g
Radix Rubiae	9 g
Crinis Carbonisatus	9 g
Pollen Typhae	9 g
Radix Salviae Miltiorrhizae	30 g
Flos Lonicerae	24 g
Semen Coicis	30 g
Bombyx Batryticatus	9 g

All the above drugs are to be decocted in water for oral administration.

Modification: For dark red bleeding, omit *Radix Rehmanniae* and *Cortex Moutan Radicis*, add 9 g of *Semen Persicae* and *Flos Carthami* each. For insufficiency of both *qi* and *blood*, add 15 g of *Radix Angelicae Sinensis* and 30 g of *Radix Astragali seu Hedysari*. For insufficiency of the spleen, add 18 g of *Radix Pseudostellariae* and 9 g of *Rhizoma Atractylodis Macrocephalae*.

Chinese Patent Medicine

Sanqi pian. Take 3 – 6 tablets each time, twice a day.

Gui pi wan. Take one bolus each time, twice a day.

Liu wei dihuang wan. Take one bolus each time, three times a day.

2. External Treatment

1) Aerosol inhalation: Refer to *Chronic Laryngitis*.
2) Avoid making sound and put the throat at rest.

Acupuncture and Moxibustion

Select two points each time from the following:
Rénying(ST9), Shuǐtū(ST10), Qūchí(LI11), Fēngchí(GB20), etc.

The treatment is given once every day with the needles retained for 30 minutes.

Chapter Twenty
Cricoarytenoid Arthritis

Cricoarytenoid arthritis is one of the chronic rheumatic arthritides of the laryngeal small joints. Its main clinical symptoms are low voice, hoarseness, pain in articulation and a sensation of obstruction in swallowing. It belongs in traditional Chinese medicine to the category of "Bì zhèng", referring to arthralgia – syndrome.

ETIOLOGY AND PATHOGENESIS

Cricoarytenoid joint is the opening and closing axis of the glottis. The disease is related to insufficiency of both *qi* and *blood* and weakened defending *qi* of the lung which result in the invasion of pathogenic wind – dampness, blocking of vessels and collaterals and stagnation of *qi* and *blood* circulation.

MAIN SYMPTOMS AND SIGNS

1. Low voice speaking, tiredness of speaking, speaking too much with a painful sensation in the throat, or hoarseness.
2. Discomfort due to burning heat in the throat, a feeling of obstruction or pain in swallowing.
3. Redness and swelling of the cricoarytenoid mucosa, dysraphism of the glottis which looks like a long triangulate crack or a triangular crack with a smaller back end. The back end of the glottis inclines to the affected part.
4. The back margin of lamina cartilaginis thyroideae may be tender.
5. At the early stage there may be fever due to aversion of cold, and sore-

ness and discomfort of the limbs.

6. Pale reddish tongue with thin and yellow fur, taut and slippery pulse.

MAIN POINTS OF DIAGNOSIS

1. The voice of the patient cannot be raised. He or she easily get tired in articulation and has difficulty in making high pitch voices. He has a pain or hoarse voice when speaking too much.

2. The patient has a feeling of fullness, dryness and pain in the throat or a sensation of obstruction when swallowing.

3. The patient has redness and swelling in the mucous membrane of the arytenoid region. It may be the same with the aryepiglottic folds and ventricular bands but the vocal cords are normal in color. The posterior end of the glottis may be inclined to the affected side. The glottis cannot get completely closed, often leaving a long triangular or a small gap at the posterior end.

4. If the joints of the two sides are affected simultaneously, difficulty in breathing may be present when the two vocal cords are abducted.

5. There is tenderness at the posterior border of the thyroid cartilage of the affected side.

6. Electrolaryngostroboscope examination indicates the presence of the vibration waves of the vocal cords.

DIFFERENTIATION AND TREATMENT OF COMMON SYNDROMES

1. Internal Treatment

Main Symptoms and Signs: There is in the throat a feeling of burning heat and a sensation of foreign body. The voice is hoarse and a pain in larynx occurs in articulation. Articulation cannot last long and high − pitch voice cannot be easily made. There is redness and swelling in the arytenoid membrane. The glottis is slant and unable to get completely closed. There are accompanying symptoms such as aversion to cold, fever and soreness in the joints of libs. The tongue is red, with yellow fur, and the pulse is taut and rapid.

Therapeutic Principles: Disperse pathogenic wind, remove dampness and regulate the functioning of the joints.

Recipe: *Decoction of ledebouriella*

Rhizoma seu Radix Notopterygii	9 g
Radix Ledebouriellae	9 g
Radix Scutellariae	9 g
Semen Armeniacae Amarum	9 g
Ramulus Cinnamomi	9 g
Radix Gentianae Macrophyllae	15 g
Radix Angelicae Sinensis	15 g
Poria	15 g
Radix Puerariae	12 g
Radix Glycyrrhizae	6 g

All the above drugs are to be decocted in water for oral administration.

Modification: For those with sore throat, add 15 grams of *Radix Clematidis*, 9 grams of *Periostracum Cicadae* and 9 grams of *Rhizoma Curcumae Longae*. For those with severe swelling in the arytenoid region, add 30 grams of *Semen Coicis* and 15 grams of *Rhizoma Alismatis*. For those who have severe redness and swelling, add 30 grams of *Caulis Lonicerae* and 15 grams of *Fructus Forsythiae*. For those who have short breath and hypodynamia, add 18 grams of *Radix Astragali seu Hedysari* and 9 grams of *Rhizoma Atractylodis Macrocephalae*.

Chinese Patent Medicine

Duhuo jisheng wan. To be taken with warm boiled water three times daily, 30 pills each time.

Qu feng zhi tong pian. Take 6 tablets each time, twice daily.

2. External Treatment

1) Compress. Use *Musk adhesive plaster for treating traumatic injury and rheumatalgia* for compress on both sides of thyroid cartilage or onto chosen points. Once daily.

2) Exercise on he cricoarytenoid joint: Pinch the laryngeal protuberance between the thumb and the index finger and shake rapidly the larynx from one side

to another, and at the same time do gentle articulation, and it is desirable to have the voice vibrate. This is done once a day, half an hour each time.

3) At the late stage, if the joint is immobilized, an operation is needed to have the immobilization removed.

Acupuncture and Moxibustion

Select two to three points from **Fútū(LI18)**, **Rényíng(ST9)**, **Shuǐtū(ST10)**, **Tiāntū(RN22)**, **Hégǔ(LI4)** and **Zhàohǎi(KI6)**. The points are punctured and the treatment is given once every other day.

Place the ignited moxa cone on a piece of ginger which is covered on the point **Rényíng(ST9)**. 5 to 7 cones can be used for each treatment.

MASSAGE

Apply massage on **Rényíng(ST9)** and **Shuǐtū(ST10)** until there is a warm feeling. The treatment is given once a day.

Part Three   Aural Diseases

Chapter One
Acute Catarrhal Otitis Media

*A*cute catarrhal otitis media is also named *acute non - suppurative otitis media* and *otitis media serosa*. It is developed from acute obstruction of tuba acustica, clinically characterized by distending and stuffy sensation in the ear, tinnitus, decrease of hearing ability, otalgia, etc.. It belongs to the category of "Ěr zhàng tòng" in traditional Chinese medicine.

ETIOLOGY AND PATHOGENESIS

It is related to blockage of the clear orifice and stagnation of meridian qi caused by ascension of the mixture of invaded pathogenic wind, heat and damp evils, and of stagnant heat due to obstructive flow of meridian qi in the liver and gallbladder.

MAIN SYMPTOMS AND SIGNS

1. Stuffy ear, decrease of hearing ability, but relieved for a moment in blowing the nose, sneezing and yawning.
2. Sensitivity to self voice.
3. Tinnitus, ear pain and symptoms of upper respiratory infection.
4. Congestion, collapse and restricted activity of tympanic membrane. If

there is accumulation of fluid in tympanic cavity, it is possible to detect liquid surface.

5. Audiometry shows conduction deafness.

MAIN POINTS OF DIAGNOSIS

1. Most of the patients have a recent history of upper respiratory tract infection.

2. The patient has a feeling of fullness in the ear as if it was stopped up with cotton and the sound seems to be farther away than it actually is. A slight earache may occur occasionally. When the patient blows the nose, there will be some change in the above – mentioned symptoms. If there is effusion in the tympanic cavity, the patient's hearing will be improved when he changes the position of the head or lies in the lateral recumbent position.

3. There are often such symptoms as autophony and infrasonic tinnitus in some cases.

4. The tympanic membrane invaginates or turns reddish. Its movement may be limited. If there is effusion in the tympanic cavity, fluid level can be seen. When the patient holds his breath to let the air enter the tympanic cavity, small bubbles can be observed.

5. The hearing test shows sound conduction hypoacusis.

DIFFERENTIATION AND TREATMENT OF COMMON SYNDROMES

1. Internal Treatment

1) **wind – cold type**

Main Symptoms and Signs: Sudden stuffy ear, ear distention and obstruction, decrease of hearing ability, hypoacusis to self voice, low – pitch tinnitus, slight red color in tympanic membrane, accompanied by severe aversion to cold, slight fever, clear nasal discharge, pale tongue, white tongue coating, superficial and tense pulse.

Therapeutic Principles: Expel wind and disperse cold for opening the orifice.

Recipe: *Jing fang bai du san*

Herba Schizonepetae	9 g
Radix Ledebouriellae	9 g
Rhizoma seu Radix Notopterygii	9 g
Radix Angelicae Pubescentis	9 g
Radix Bupleuri	12 g
Radix Platycodi	6 g
Rhizoma Ligustici Chuanxiong	9 g
Radix Angelicae Dahuricae	15 g
Flos Magnoliae	9 g
Caulis Akebiae	6 g
Rhizoma Acori Graminei	9 g
Radix Glycyrrhizae	6 g

All the above drugs are to be decocted in water for oral administration.

Recipe: *Jia wei xin yi san*

Flos Magnoliae	9 g
Radix Ledebouriellae	9 g
Rhizoma Ligustici Chuanxiong	9 g
Rhizoma Cimicifugae	9 g
Frucus Xanthii	9 g
Rhizoma Acori Graminei	9 g
Rhizoma et Radix Ligustici	12 g
Radix Angelicae Dahuricae	18 g
Caulis Akebiae	6 g
Herba Asari	3 g
Radix Glycyrrhizae	3 g

All the above drugs are to be decocted in water for oral administration.

2) **wind – heat type**

Main Symptoms and Signs: Sudden stuffy ear, distention and blockage in the ear, like stuffed with cotton, decrease of hearing ability, hypoacusis to self voice, tinnitus of low frequency, congestion in tympanic membrane with disappearance of normal landmarks, conduction deafness in the sick ear, redness and swelling of nasal mucous membrane, tenacious nasal discharge, accompanied by slight aversion to cold and wind, high fever, sore throat, turbid nasal discharge, red tongue, thin and yellow tongue coating, superficial and rapid pulse.

Therapeutic Principles: Expel wind and clarify heat for opening the orifice and benefiting hearing ability.

Recipe: *Yin qiao san*

Flos Lonicerae	15 g
Fructus Forsythiae	12 g
Herba Schizonepetae	9 g
Herba Menthae	6 g
Fructus Arctii	9 g
Radix Platycodi	9 g
Rhizoma Ligustici Chuanxiong	9 g
Radix Scutellariae	9 g
Rhizoma Acori Graminei	9 g
Caulis Akebiae	6 g
Radix Glycyrrhizae	6 g

All the above drugs are to be decocted in water for oral administration.

Modification: For turbid nasal discharge, add 9 g of *Frucus Xanthii* and 9 g of *Rhizoma Paridis*. For cough and excessive sputum, add 9 g of *Rhizoma Pinelliae* and 9 g of *Semen Armeniacae Amarum*. For accumulated fluid in the orifice, add 9 g of *Rhizoma Alismatis*, 15 g of *Semen Plantaginis* and 30 g of *Semen Coicis*.

Chinese Patent Medicine

Ling yang gan mao pian. Take 6 tablets each time, 3 times daily.

3) accumulation of dampness in the ear

Main Symptoms and Signs: The patient has a feeling of fullness and obstruction in the ear, tinnitus which is like the chirping of cicadas, deafness and the sound he hears seems to be farther away than it actually is. If the patient changes the position of his or her head or lies in the lateral recumbent position, the hearing will improve. The drum membrane invaginates and looks red. Fluid level or bubbles can be seen in the tympanic cavity. There may be accompanying sensation of heaviness in the head, aversion to wind and poor appetite. The fur is white and greasy and the pulse is soft and slippery.

Therapeutic Principles: Remove pathogenic dampness and obstruction from the upper orifices.

Recipe: *Diuretic powder of four drugs*

Polyporus	15 g
Rhizoma Alismatis	15 g
Rhizoma Atractylodis Macrocephalae	9 g
Herba Asari	3 g
Rhizoma Acori Graminei	12 g
Flos Lonicerae	30 g

All the above drugs are to be decocted in water for oral administration.

Modification: For those who have headache and stuffy nose, add 9 grams of *Rhizoma Ligustici Chuanxiong* and 9 grams of *Fructus Viticis*. For those who have deficiency of the spleen manifested as poor appetite, add 30 grams of *Semen Coicis*, 9 grams of *Pericarpium Citri Reticulatae* and 9 grams of *Fructus Amomi*.

2. External Treatment

1) Nasal drip with *Di bi ling*. The ingredients is as follows:

Herba Centipedae	650 g
Flos Magnoliae	150 g

First decoct the drugs in water twice, then mix the two decoctions and concentrate the mixture into 1,500 ml of solution. Add 3.75 grams of **powder of ephedrine hydrochloride** and 15 grams of **powder of glucose** into the solution and, after filtration and sterilization, put the solution into a bottle for nasal drip, which should be done 3 times a day.

2) Ear drip with **herbal auristilla** which is prepared and used as follows:

Have some *Herba Saxifragae* pounded into a jelly, squeeze it, get the juice, add a small amount of *Borneolum Syntheticum* into the juice and drip it into the ear, three times a day.

3) Press tragus with the tip of small finger, or insert the tip of small finger into the external auditory canal. Do the pressing and relaxing repeatedly.

Acupuncture and Moxibustion

Select 3 to 5 points from **Tīnggōng(SI19)**, **Tīnghuì(GB2)**, **Yìfēng(SJ17)**, **Fēngchí(GB20)**, **Nèiguān(PC6)** and **Hégǔ(LI4)**. Puncture the points and retain the needles for 20 minutes.

Chapter Two
Chronic Catarrhal Otitis Media

Chronic catarrhal otitis media (chronic non-suppurative otitis media) is a chronic non-suppurative inflammation of the mucous membrane of the eustachian tube and middle ear cavity, mostly due to the inappropriate treatment of acute otitis media. Its clinical characteristics are a feeling of fullness in the ear, hard hearing and long duration. it falls into the category of "ěr bì" (ear plug) or "ěr lóng" (deafness) in traditional Chinese medicine.

ETIOLOGY AND PATHOGENESIS

It is due to *yin* insufficiency in the kidney, or *qi* deficiency in the lung and spleen which fails to transport essence of water and grain upwards to the orifice of the ear, causing accumulation of evils, stagnation of *qi* and *blood* stasis, disharmony between ying and wei, and hence resulting in *qi* stagnation and accumulation of evils.

MAIN SYMPTOMS AND SIGNS

1. Ear stuffiness, ear distention which is like stuffed with cotton.
2. Decrease of hearing ability, conduction deafness at the initial stage, mixture deafness at the late stage, low-pitch tinnitus which often changes in blowing the nose.
3. Tympanic membrane becomes collapsed, thickened, or thinner, even calcified, and adhesive.
4. Frequent recurrence and comparative long duration.

MAIN POINTS OF DIAGNOSIS

1. It occurs mostly in adults.
2. The patient has a sensation of fullness and oppression in the ear. The hypoacusis gradually becomes severer and severer, and it is latent in nature. Paracusia Willisiana may be present. may be present. The hearing test shows sound-conducting deafness at the initial stage and mixed deafness at the late stage.
3. The tinnitus is low-pitched or intermittent.
4. The drum membrane invaginates, becoming thick or atrophic with adhesion and calcareous deposits on it.

DIFFERENTIATION AND TREATMENT OF COMMON SYNDROMES

1. Internal Treatment

Main Symptoms and Signs: The patient has a feeling of fullness in the ear, hard hearing, and droning tinnitus. The drum membrane invaginates and looks turbid, with its movement limited, accompanied by dizziness and malaise, light red tongue and thready and feeble pulse.

Therapeutic Principles: Promote the flow of *qi* and *blood* circulation and remove obstruction from the upper orifices

Recipe: *Decoction for activating blood circulation* compounded with *Powder for promoting the flow of qi*

Semen Persicae	9 g
Flos Carthami	9 g
Rhizoma Ligustici Chuanxiong	9 g
Rhizoma Zingiberis Recens	9 g
Radix Bupleuri	9 g
Radix Paeoniae Rubra	9 g
Rhizoma Cyperi	9 g
Bulbus Allii Fistulosi	3 pcs
Fructus Ziziphi Jujubae	7 pcs
Moschus	150 mg

millet wine   250 ml

Decoct the first 9 ingredients in water and discharge the dregs. Wrap the musk in a piece of cloth and put it into the wine which is to be boiled twice or three times. Mix the above two decoctions and take the mixture before bedtime. The musk can be used repeatedly.

Modification: For those who have constant tinnitus, add 9 grams of *Rhizoma Cibotii*, 15 grams of *Semen Cuscutae* and 30 grams of *Magnetitum*. For those who are deficient in the liver and kidney, *Kidney − yin − reinforcing bolus* is also to be taken at the same time. For fluid accumulation in the middle ear, add 15 g of *Semen Plantaginis*, 15 g of *Rhizoma Alismatis* and 30 g of *Semen Coicis*. For poor appetite, abdominal distention and loose stool, add 15 g of *Radix Codonopsis Pilosulae*, 12 g of *Radix Astragali seu Hedysari*, 12 g of *Radix Angelicae Sinensis*. For cold sensation in the body and limbs, pale facial complexion, add 9 g of *Ramulus Cinnamomi* and 9 g of *Radix Aconiti Praeparata*.

2. External Treatment

It is advisable to put 3 to drops of *Di bi ling* and *Xinyi you di bi ling* into the nose each time, 3 to 4 times a day.

Acupuncture and Moxibustion

Select 2 to 4 points from **Hégǔ(LI4)**, **Tīnggōng(SI19)**, **Tīnghuì(GB2)**, **Ěrmén(SJ21)**, **Yìfēng(SJ17)** and **Zúsānlǐ(ST36)**. The needles are retained for 20 minutes. Once daily.

Chapter Three
Acute Suppurative Otitis Media

Acute suppurative otitis media refers to acute infection caused by invasion of suppurative bacteria in mucous membrane and periost of the middle ear. Clinically it is characterized by ear pain, fever, and ps effusion in the ear. It is similar to the category of "shí zhèng nóng ěr" (suppurative ear of excessive type) in traditional Chinese medicine. It is a commonly seen in otology and often happens in children.

ETIOLOGY AND PATHOGENESIS

It is due to invasion of pathogenic wind and heat evils which go to the ear through meridians, and causes accumulation of heat – toxin, and hence the accumulated heat steams and burns tympanic membrane, resulting in decay of blood and flesh and in turn perforation of tympanic membrane; or it is due to the affection of exogenous pathogenic factors, emotional factors and fire created from stagnation of liver qi which are sent upward to the ear orifice along the *Gallbladder Meridian*, resulting in the mixture of the external and internal evils, and hence causing suppuration and perforation in tympanic membrane.

MAIN SYMPTOMS AND SIGNS

1. Ear pain, even throbbing pain, is progressively aggravated so that sleeping often would be influenced. As soon as tympanic membrane perforates or is incised, ear pain and body temperature would be relieved and decreased markedly.

2. Accompanied by high fever, aversion to cold, headache and uncomfortable sensation in the whole body.

3. Conductive decrease of hearing ability, accompanied by tinnitus.

4. Local or diffuse congestion in tympanic membrane, or external prominence of tympanic membrane can be noticed. At the initial stage, perforating in pars tensa of tympanic membrane is small, with flashing and throbbing pus effusion which is in bloody fluid at the beginning and in purulence at the later stage, hence perforation enlarges.

MAIN POINTS OF DIAGNOSIS

1. This disease is in most cases caused by upper respiratory tract infection or the dirty water which gets into the ear, most often seen at the end of winter and the beginning of spring as well as in summer. Infants are especially vulnerable to this disease.

2. There is pain in the ear. In severe cases, a throbbing pain my be present. After pus is discharged from the ear, the pain is relieved.

3. Pus comes out from the ear, at first white in color or with a little blood in it, and then yellow, thick and profuse pus runs out.

4. At the early stage the drum membrane is marked by diffuse hyperemia, looking bright red or dull red and bulging. Then perforation of tympanic membrane appears with pus running out. If the pus cannot get out easily, a pulsating discharge may be seen. If the hole is big, the pus will gush out.

5. The tinnitus is of low pitch and the deafness sound - conductive. \ ;6. The patient may have a fever, headache and stuffy and running nose. Infant cases or patients of children may keep crying and be unquiet. The infantile patients may refuse to suck.

DIFFERENTIATION AND TREATMENT OF COMMON SYNDROMES

1. Internal Treatment

1) **invasion of the ear by exopathic wind - heat toxin**

Main Symptoms and Signs: The patient has otalgia and a feeling of fullness in the ear. There is white or yellow pus coming out from it. Perforation of membrana tensa appears and from it pus comes out in pulsation, also accompanied by aversion to cold, fever, headache and stuffy nose. The infantile patients may keep crying and unquiet. The fur of the tongue is thin and white and the pulse floating and rapid.

Therapeutic Principles: Disperse pathogenic wind and heat and remove toxin to relieve swelling.

Recipe: *Powder of lonicera and forsythia*, compounded with *xanthium powder*

Flos Lonicerae	30 g
Fructus Forsythiae	15 g
Rhizoma Phragmitis	15 g
Herba Menthae	9 g
Herba Lophatheri	9 g
Semen Sojae Praeparatum	9 g
Fructus Arctii	9 g
Frucus Xanthii	9 g
Flos Magnoliae	9 g
Herba Schizonepetae	12 g
Radix Angelicae Dahuricae	18 g
Radix Glycyrrhizae	6 g

All the above drugs are to be decocted in water for oral administration.

Recipe: *Yin qiao san* et *Wu wei xiao du yin* jia jian

Flos Lonicerae	15 g
Fructus Forsythiae	9 g
Herba Menthae	6 g
Fructus Arctii	9 g
Herba Schizonepetae	9 g
Herba Taraxaci	15 g
Herba Violae	15 g
Flos Chrysanthemi Indici	15 g
Rhizoma Phragmitis	15 g
Radix Platycodi	9 g
Fructus Liquidambaris	9 g
Radix Glycyrrhizae	6 g

All the above drugs are to be decocted in water for oral administration.

Modification: For nasal discharge and obstruction, add 6 g of *Stigma Maydis*. For headache, add 9 g of *Herba Artemisiae Chinghao* and 3 g of *Herba Asari*.

Chinese Patent Medicine

Xi ling jie du wan. Take one pill each time, twice a day.

2) damp - heat in the liver and gallbladder

Main Symptoms and Signs: There is a severe jumping pain in the ear which may radiate to the head. A yellow and thick pus comes out of the ear. A big perforation of the membrana tensa occurs and the pus gushes out, accompanied by a hypoacusis, a bitter taste and a dry throat, red tongue with yellow and greasy fur, and taut and rapid pulse.

Therapeutic Principles: Clear away pathogenic heat from the liver and gallbladder and remove dampness and pus.

Recipe: *Decoction of gentian for purging liver - fire*

Radix Gentianae	9 g
Radix Scutellariae	9 g
Radix Bupleuri	9 g
Fructus Gardeniae	15 g
Radix Angelicae Sinensis	15 g
Radix Rehmanniae	15 g
Rhizoma Alismatis	15 g
Semen Plantaginis	15 g
Radix Glycyrrhizae	6 g
Caulis Akebiae	6 g

All the above drugs are to be decocted in water for oral administration.

Modification: For those who have pain in he ear and difficulty for the pus to come out, add 9 grams of *Spina Gleditsiae*, 9 grams of *Squama Manitis*. For those with profuse pus, add 15 grams of *Fructus Kochiae*, 9 grams of *Radix Sophorae Flavescentis* and 30 grams of *Radix Trichosanthis*. For those who have constipation, add 9 grams of *Radix et Rhizoma Rhei* and 9 grams of *Natrii Sulphas*. For restless infants, add 6 grams of *Periostracum Cicadae* and 6 grams of *Ramulus Uncariae cum Uncis* which is to be decocted later than other drugs. For infantile nausea, add 4.5 g of *Concretio Siliceae Bambusae* and 6 g of *Caulis Bambusae in Taeniam*.

Chinese Patent Medicine

Long dan xie gan wan. Take 6 g each time, twice a day.

2. External Treatment

1) **Clean pus**: Dip cotton stick in dilute vinegar (edible vinegar added with proportional cold boiled water) and wash out pus.

2) **Drop ear**: Choose *Huanglian di er ye*, *Yu xing cao di er ye* and *Xuan shen di er ye* to put 2 to 3 drops into the ear each time, 3 to 4 times a day. It is also suitable to smash fresh *Herba Saxifragae* or fresh *Folium Mori* to extract juice for dropping the ear with above-mentioned method.

Acupuncture and Moxibustion

Select 3 to 5 points from **Tīnggōng(SI19)**, **Tīnghuì(GB2)**, **Yìfēng(SJ17)**, **Qīuxū(GB40)**, **Ěrmén(SJ21)**, **Yánglíngquán(GB34)**, **Xiáxī(GB43)**, **Qūchí(LI11)**, **Wàiguān(SJ5)** and **Hégǔ(LI4)**. Retain the needles for 20 minutes. The treatment is given once every day.

Ignite one side of a moxa-stick and heat **Yìfēng(SJ17)** one inch away from the acupoint till the skin feels hot and becomes red and wet. One treatment is given every day.

Chapter Four
Sudden Deafness

*S*udden deafness, a sensorineural hearing loss, occurs abruptly for reasons unknown. Its main clinical feature is a sudden profound sensorineural deafness, accompanied by tinnitus and dizziness and a tendency to get cured spontaneously. The disorder is usually unilateral and occurs more often in females and mostly in the middle-aged. In traditional Chinese medicine, it belongs to the category of "Bào lóng" or "Cù lóng", both meaning sudden deafness.

ETIOLOGY AND PATHOGENESIS

It is elated to invasion of external pathogenic wind and internal injury of seven emotional factors, which causes stagnation of meridians in the ear orifice, disharmony between *qi* and *blood*.

MAIN POINTS OF DIAGNOSIS

1. In some cases there exist mental factors or a history of virus infection prior to the attack of the disease.
2. It occurs abruptly. The patient often has severe deafness or even loses hearing entirely within an hour or one day.
3. There is often an accompanying tinnitus or vertigo.
4. Otic endoscopy examination indicates normal.
5. Audiometric curve shows that the deafness is a sensorineural hearing loss. Low-frequency deafness and even deafness are seen more often and recruitment may be present.

DIFFERENTIATION AND TREATMENT OF COMMON SYNDROMES

1. Internal Treatment

Main Symptoms and Signs: Deafness and tinnitus suddenly occur, in most cases resulting from tense mood or overwork, and are accompanied with restlessness, irritability, dizziness, and insomnia. The tongue is light red with little fur. The pulse is taut.

Therapeutic Principles: Promoting the flow of *qi* and *blood* circulation, relaxing muscles and tendons and removing obstruction from the channels.

Recipe: *Decoction for Activating Blood Circulation with additional drugs*

Semen Persicae	9 g
Flos Carthami	9 g
Rhizoma Ligustici Chuanxiong	9 g
Rhizoma Acori Graminei	9 g
Radix Bupleuri	9 g
Radix Paeoniae Rubra	15 g
Bombyx Batryticatus	9 g
Radix Salviae Miltiorrhizae	15 g
Radix Puerariae	15 g
Allium Fistulosum	3 stems
Radix Paeoniae Rubra	9 g
Radix Puerariae	30 g
Rhizoma Zingiberis Recens	6 g
Fructus Ziziphi Jujubae	7 pcs
Moschus (ground and taken with water)	20 mg

Modification: For those who have a feeling of fullness and discomfort in the chest and hypochondrium as well as restlessness and irritability, add 9 grams of *gentian root*, 9 grams of *scutellaria root* and 15 grams of *capejasmine fruit*. For those with severe tinnitus, add 30 grams of *magnetite* which is to be decocted first and 9 grams of *chastetree fruit*. For those with dizziness, add 30 grams of *fleece-flower stem*, 9 grams of *gastrodia tuber* and 30 grams of *abalone shell*. For those accompanied y fullness and stuffiness in the chest and hypochondria, distention in the head, headache, flushed cheeks, red eyes, frustration, irritability, red tongue, yellow tongue coating, and wiry pulse, add *Radix Scutellariae* 9 g and *Rhizoma Alismatis* 9 g. For stuffiness and distention in the ear, add *Fructus Viticis* 9 g, *Flos Chrysanthemi* 9 g, *Rhizoma Cimicifugae* 6 g. For vertigo, add *Os Draconis* 30 g, *Concha Ostreae* 30 g and *Concha Margaitifera Usta* 30 g.

Chinese Patent Medicine

Fufang danshen pian. Take 2 tablets each time, 3 times a day. *Longdan xie gan wan*. Take 6 g each time, twice a day.

2. External Treatment

Recipe:

Herba Asari	7.5 g
Rhizoma Acori Graminei	7.5 g
Semen Armeniacae Amarum	13 g
Massa Fermentata	13 g

Pound them and make into bolus of jujubecore-size, and put the bolus packaged with silkfloss into the external auditory canal, and change the bolus once every day. After it is effective the bolus can be taken once every other day.

Acupuncture and Moxibustion

The points are **Yìfēng(SJ17)**, **Tīnggōng(SI19)**, **Tīnghuì(GB2)**, **Ěrmén(SJ21)**, **Zhōngzhǔ(SJ3)**, **Wàiguān(SJ5)**, **Yánglíngquán(GB34)**, **Xiáxī(GB43)**, **Sānyīnjiāo(SP6)** and **Zúsānlǐ(ST36)**. 3 to 4 points among them are selected each time. Reducing method. The treatment is given once daily.

Injection therapy may also be applied. 2 ml of *Danshen zhusheye* or *Danggui zhusheye* is injected into **Yìfēng(SJ17)** and **Tīnggōng(SI19)**. The treatment is given once every other day, ten treatments as one course.

Chapter Five
Senile Deafness

Senile deafness refers to the progressive decrease of hearing ability on both ears after middle age and it is often related to heredity. Clinically it is characterized by bilateral, chronic and progressive deafness, and it belongs to the category of "Shèn xū ěr lóng" (deafness due to kidney deficiency) in traditional Chinese medicine.

ETIOLOGY AND PATHOGENESIS

Kidney opens into the ears and kidney qi flows into the ears. Only when essence and qi in the kidney are sufficient and plentiful, and when the source of bone marrow is nourished, can the hearing ability be sensitive, and can the distinguishing powder be higher. In the senile cases, essence and qi in the kidney start to subside, resulting in decrease of the hearing ability.

MAIN SYMPTOMS AND SIGNS

1. It often starts after 50 years old, the hearing ability decreases progressively, and especially hearing ability of high frequency decreases first.
2. The decrease of the hearing abilities symmetrical on both sides, diagnosed as nervous deafness without vibration.
3. The tympanic membrane looks grey, dark and lustrousless in color.

DIFFERENTIATION AND TREATMENT OF COMMON SYNDROMES

1. Internal Treatment

1) insufficiency of kidney essence

Main Symptoms and Signs: Progressive decrease of the hearing ability in both ears, accompanied by soft tinnitus which is relieved in the morning and aggravated in the evening, decrease in mentality, slow in action weakness in feet, spermatorrhea, impotence, pale tongue, scanty tongue coating, thready and rapid pulse.

Therapeutic Principles: Nourish the kidney, replenish essence and relieve deafness.

Recipe: *Er long zuo ci tang*

Radix Rehmanniae Praeparata	15 g
Rhizoma Dioscoreae	15 g
Fructus Corni	15 g
Poria	24 g
Rhizoma Alismatis	12 g
Cortex Moutan Radicis	9 g
Magnetitum	30 g
Fructus Schisandrae	6 g
Rhizoma Acori Graminei	9 g

All the above drugs are to be decocted in water for oral administration.

Modification: For aggravated tinnitus at night, add 9 g of *Semen Juglandis*, 9 g of *Fructus Psoraleae* and 9 g of *Semen Cuscutae*. For dizziness and blurring of vision, add 9 g of *Concha Haliotidis* and 9 g of *Semen Celosiae*. For feverish sensation in the palms and soles, and insomnia, add 15 g of *Cortex Lycii Radicis* and 15 g of *Cortex Mori Radicis*.

Chinese Patent Medicine

Er long zuo ci wan. Take 9 grams each time, twice a day.

2) deficiency of kidney *qi*

Main Symptoms and Signs: Progressive deafness, slight tinnitus, accompanied by shortness of breath due to exertion, loose stool, urine in large volume, enuresis, dribbling of urine, pale tongue with white coating, deep and feeble pulse.

Therapeutic Principles: Tonify the kidney, benefit qi and relieve deafness.

Recipe: *You gui yin*

Radix Rehmanniae Praeparata	15 g
Rhizoma Dioscoreae	15 g
Fructus Corni	15 g
Fructus Lycii	9 g
Colla Cornus Cervi	6 g
Semen Cuscutae	15 g
Cortex Eucommiae	9 g
Radix Angelicae Sinensis	12 g
Cortex Cinnamomi	9 g
Radix Aconiti Praeparata	9 g

All the above drugs are to be decocted in water for oral administration.

Modification: For shortness of breath due to exertion, add 9 g of *Fructus Psoraleae* and 3 g of *Gecko*. For tinnitus, add 30 g of *Magnetitum* and 9 g of *Rhizoma Acori Graminei*. For abdominal distention and fullness, add 30 g of *Semen Coicis* and 12 g of *Rhizoma Alismatis*.

Chinese Patent Medicine

You gui wan. Take one pill each time, 3 times a day.

Acupuncture and Moxibustion

Select 3 to 5 points from **Ěrmén (SJ21)**, **Tīnghuì (GB2)**, **Yìfēng (SJ17)**, **Zhōngzhǔ(SJ3)**, **Wàiguān(SJ5)**, **Yánglíngquán(GB34)**, **Zúsānlǐ(ST36)** and **Sānyīnjiāo (SP6)**. Retain the needles for 30 minutes to one hour. The treatment is given once a day.

Chapter Six
Nervous Tinnitus

Nervous tinnitus refers to the disease characterized clinically by high – pitch tinnitus and without dysfunction in the hearing ability, and it belongs to the category of "Ěr lóng" in traditional Chinese medicine.

ETIOLOGY AND PATHOGENESIS

It is mostly related to insufficiency of kidney – *yin* and ascension of deficient *fire* which disturb the clear orifice, or is related to deficiency and consumption of meridians around the eyes and ears, or ascension of liver *fire* which disturbs upwards the clear orifice, and causing tinnitus.

MAIN SYMPTOMS AND SIGNS

1. Continuous high – pitch tinnitus, aggravated at night.
2. Mostly, subjective tinnitus.
3. Mostly, normal hearing ability.
3. Normal or slight collapse in tympanic membrane.

DIFFERENTIATION AND TREATMENT OF COMMON SYNDROMES

Internal Treatment

1) **insufficiency of kidney – *yin***

Main Symptoms and Signs: Slight and continuous tinnitus in cicada's chirp, aggravated at night, feverish sensation in the palms and soles, soreness and weakness in the low back and knees, dizziness and blurring of vision, red tongue, scanty tongue coating, thready and rapid pulse.

Therapeutic Principles: Tonify *yin*, subside *fire* and stop tinnitus.

Recipe: *Zhi bai di huang tang*

Rhizoma Anemarrhenae	9 g
Cortex Phellodendri	9 g
Fructus Corni	30 g
Rhizoma Dioscoreae	30 g
Poria	18 g
Rhizoma Alismatis	12 g
Cortex Moutan Radicis	9 g
Radix Rehmanniae Praeparata	
Magnetitum	
Concha Ostreae	30 g

All the above drugs are to be decocted in water for oral administration.

Modification: For tinnitus aggravated at night and luxation of teeth, add 15 g of *Semen Juglandis* and 15 g of *Fluoritum*.

Chinese Patent Medicine

Zhi bai dihuang wan. Take one pill each time, twice a day.

2) deficiency in the heart and spleen

Main Symptoms and Signs: Deficient tinnitus, aggravated by fatigue and standing up from squat, lustrousless facial complexion, palpitation, insomnia, pale lips, pale tongue, thin and white tongue coating, thready and weak pulse.

Therapeutic Principles: Tonify and benefit the heart and spleen.

Recipe: *Gui pi tang*

Rhizoma Atractylodis Macrocephalae	9 g
Poria cum Ligno Hospite	9 g
Radix Astragali seu Hedysari	12 g
Arillus Longan	12 g
Semen Ziziphi Spinosae	30 g
Radix Codonopsis Pilosulae	15 g
Radix Glycyrrhizae Praeparata	9 g

Radix Angelicae Sinensis	12 g
Radix Polygalae	9 g
Radix Aucklandiae	9 g
Magnetitum	30 g
Rhizoma Zingiberis Recens	3 slices
Fructus Ziziphi Jujubae	5 pieces

All the above drugs are to be decocted in water for oral administration.

Chinese Patent Medicine

Gui pi wan. Take one pill each time, twice a day.

3) **ascension of liver** *fire*

Main Symptoms and Signs: Loud tinnitus, aggravated by emotional disturbance, accompanied by headache, ear pain, flushed cheeks, red eyes, distending pain in the chest and hypochondria, red tongue, yellow tongue coating, wiry and rapid pulse.

Therapeutic Principles: Clear the liver and subside *fire*.

Recipe: *Dan zhi xiao yao san*

Radix Bupleuri	15 g
Radix Angelicae Sinensis	12 g
Radix Paeoniae Alba	15 g
Rhizoma Atractylodis Macrocephalae	9 g
Poria	15 g
Herba Menthae	9 g
Cortex Moutan Radicis	9 g
Fructus Gardeniae	9 g
Fructus Liquidambaris	9 g
Concha Ostreae	30 g
Rhizoma Zingiberis Recens	3 slices
Radix Glycyrrhizae	6 g

All the above drugs are to be decocted in water for oral administration.

Modification: For otalgia, add 9 g of **Radix Saussureae Lappae** and 9 g of *Aloe*.

Chinese Patent Medicine

Long dan xie gan wan. Take 6 g each time, twice a day.

Nervous Tinnitus

Acupuncture and Moxibustion

Select 3 to 5 points from **Ěrmén**(SJ21), **Tīnggōng**(SI19), **Tīnghuì**(GB2), **Yìfēng** (SJ17), **Zhōngzhǔ**(SJ3), **Wàiguān**(SJ5), **Yánglíngquán**(GB34), **Zúsānlǐ**(ST36) and **Sānyīnjiāo**(SP6). Punctured with medium stimulation. The treatment is given once a day.

Chapter Seven
Ménière's Disease

Ménière's disease is also known as hydrops of membranous labyrinth. Its clinical characteristics are paroxysmal dizziness, fluctuating deafness, tinnitus and a feeling of fullness in the ear. It belongs to the category of "Xuàn yūn" (dizziness) in traditional Chinese medicine.

ETIOLOGY AND PATHOGENESIS

Water metabolism of the human body is associated with the lung, spleen and kidney. The spleen dominates transportation and transformation, the lung is responsible for regulating the passage for water flow, the kidney serves for warming up body fluid. The deficiency in the lung, spleen and kidney would cause dysfunction in water flow, which accumulates dampness into phlegm and then the phlegm disturbs the clear orifice upwards, resulting in dizziness. The kidney stores essence and produces bone marrow, if essence and bone marrow are insufficient, the orifice of the ear would lack nourishment, resulting in dizziness. If the liver qi is stagnant, it would turn into fire and produce wind, both of which attack the clear orifice upwards, causing dizziness.

MAIN SYMPTOMS AND SIGNS

1. Dizziness: It is described as sudden and rotatory vertigo aggravated by exertion, accompanied by nystagmus, pallor, cold sweat, nausea and vomiting, but with clear consciousness.
2. Tinnitus: It is continuous, low-frequent and low-pitch, or aggravated in attack.
3. Deafness: It is nervous deafness with vibration.
4. In attack of vertigo, it is possible to notice spontaneous nystagmus,

mostly in horizontal movement. After repeated attacks, the functions of vestibule would decrease in most cases and the tympanic membrane is normal.

MAIN POINTS OF DIAGNOSIS

1. It occurs most often in middle-aged males, as a result of fatigue, change in mood and lack of sleep.
2. The patient suffers from paroxysmal vertigo and a sensation of rotating around or floating-and-sinking, accompanied with spontaneous nystagemus, nausea, vomiting, pallor and cold sweating. The dizziness may last for several minutes or even several hours, but the patient is conscious.
3. Constant tinnitus occurs, which is aggravated before or after the attack of the disease.
4. The patient has sensorineural deafness. It fluctuates prior to and after the attack of the disease. Hyper-sensitive sign to high-pitch sound may occur.
5. The patient has a feeling of fullness in the ear and head.
6. Examination show the drum membrane is normal. There is horizontal or slightly rotatory nystagmus during the attack. Hearing test indicates a sensorineural hypoacusis and recruitment may be present. The vestibular function test shows that its function is reduced during the period of the attack.
7. Glycerin test shows positive.

DIFFERENTIATION AND TREATMENT OF COMMON SYNDROMES

1. hyperactivity of liver-yang

Main Symptoms and Signs: Vertigo occurs mostly after a change in mood. Tinnitus like chattering sound of machine is present, accompanied with restlessness, irritability, headache and a feeling of fullness in the ear as well as flushing face, red eyes, a bitter taste in the mouth and dryness in the throat. The tongue is red and its fur yellow. The pulse is taut and rapid.

Therapeutic Principles: Calming the liver to stop endogenous wind and nourishing yin to suppress yang.

Recipe: *Decoction of Gastrodia and Uncaria*

Rhizoma Gastrodiae	9 g
Radix Scutellariae	9 g
Radix Achyranthis Bidentatae	9 g
Cortex Eucommiae	9 g
Ramulus Uncariae cum Uncis (decocted later)	15 g
Fructus Gardeniae	15 g
Herba Leonuri	15 g
Ramulus Loranthi	15 g
Caulis Polygoni Multiflori	15 g
Poria cum Ligno Hospite	15 g
Concha Haliotidis (decocted first)	30 g

All the above drugs are to be decocted in water for oral administration.

Modification: For severe tinnitus, add 9 g of *Rhizoma Acori Graminei*, and 30 g of *Magnetitum*. For numbness in the extremities, add 30 g of *Os Draconis* and 30 g of *Concha Ostreae*. For hyperactivity of liver fire, add 6 g of *Radix Gentianae* and 9 g of *Cortex Moutan Radicis*. For warm sensation in the palms and soles, add 9 g of *Rhizoma Anemarrhenae* and 9 g of *Cortex Phellodendri*.

Chinese Patent Medicine

Tianma houpo wan. Take one pill each time, twice a day.

Nao li qing. Take 10 pills each time, twice a week.

2. turbid phlegm obstruction in the middle-jiao

Main Symptoms and Signs: There are such symptoms as dizziness and shakiness, which will be aggravated by movements, accompanied with nausea, vomiting, a sensation of heaviness in the head as if it were tightly wrapped up, a feeling of fullness in the chest and poor appetite. The fur of the tongue is white and greasy and the pulse taut and slippery.

Recipe: *Decoction of Pinellia, White Atractylodes and Gastrodia*

Rhizoma Pinelliae Praeparata	9 g
Rhizoma Atractylodis Macrocephalae	9 g
Rhizoma Gastrodiae	9 g
Pericarpium Citri Reticulatae	9 g
Poria cum Ligno Hospite	15 g
Radix Glycyrrhizae	6 g

Rhizoma Zingiberis Recens	6 g
Fructus Ziziphi Jujubae	7 pcs

All the above drugs are to be decocted in water for oral administration.

Modification: For severe fullness and stuffiness in the chest and epigastrium, add 9 g of *Fructus Amomi* and 9 g of *Pericarpium Citri Reticulatae*. For frequent vomiting, add 30 g of *Haematitum* and 9 g of *Flos Inulae*. For shortness of breath and lassitude, add 15 g of *Radix Astragali seu Hedysari* and 9 g of *Radix Ginseng*.

Chinese Patent Medicine

Banxia baizhu tianma wan. Take 6 g each time, twice a day. *Er chen wan*. Take 6 g each time, twice a day.

3. deficiency of both spleen and kidney

Main Symptoms and Signs: There are repeated occurrences of vertigo and tinnitus which is like singing of cicadas, accompanied with short breath, fatigue, soreness and weakness of the waist and knees, amnesia, excessive dreaming during sleep, clear urine and long - time urination at night, reddish tongue with white fur, and thready and feeble pulse.

Therapeutic Principles: Replenishing *qi*, warming the kidney and removing water retention to relieve dizziness.

Recipe: *Decoction for Reinforcing Middle - jiao and Replenishing qi*, compounded with *Diuretic Decoction by Strengthening Yang of the Spleen and Kidney*

Radix Astragali seu Hedysari	24 g
Radix Ginseng	9 g
Rhizoma Atractylodis Macrocephalae	9 g
Pericarpium Citri Reticulatae	9 g
Rhizoma Cimicifugae	9 g
Radix Bupleuri	9 g
Radix Aconiti Praeparata	9 g
Rhizoma Zingiberis Recens	9 g
Radix Angelicae Sinensis	15 g
Poria cum Ligno Hospite	15 g
Radix Paeoniae Alba	15 g
Radix Glycyrrhizae	6 g

All the above drugs are to be decocted in water for oral administration.

Modification: For those who have excessive liver-fire, add 9 grams of *Radix Gentianae* and 9 grams of *Cortex Moutan Radicis*. For those who have severe tinnitus, add 9 grams of *Magnetitum* and 9 grams of *Rhizoma Acori Graminei*. For those suffering from insomnia and dysphoria, add 15 grams of *Caulis Polygoni Multiflori*, 15 grams of *Os Draconis Fossilia Ossis Mastodi* and 15 grams of *Concha Ostreae*. For those with severe nausea and vomiting, add 15 grams of *Haematitum*, 9 grams of *Flos Inulae* (wrapped in a piece of gauze before it is decocted) and 6 grams of *Caulis Bambusae in Taeniam*.

4. deficiency of qi and blood

Main Symptoms and Signs: Vertigo accompanied by pallor and lusterless complexion, short breath, palpitation, insomnia, pale lips and nails, lassitude, pale tongue, thready and weak pulse.

Therapeutic Principles: Replenish *qi* and *blood*.

Recipe:

Radix Codonopsis Pilosulae	15 g
Radix Astragali seu Hedysari	30 g
Rhizoma Atractylodis Macrocephalae	12 g
Pericarpium Citri Reticulatae	9 g
Rhizoma Cimicifugae	9 g
Radix Bupleuri	9 g
Radix Angelicae Sinensis	12 g
Radix Paeoniae Alba	15 g
Radix Glycyrrhizae Praeparata	6 g

All the above drugs are to be decocted in water for oral administration.

Chinese Patent Medicine

Angelica blood-supplementing pill (Danggui yangxue wan). Take 9 g, twice daily.

5. upward flooding of cold water

Main Symptoms and Signs: Palpitation in the attack of vertigo, pain in low back, cold sensation in the back, cold limbs, low-spirits, cough, thin and white sputum, profuse urine, pale tongue, thin and white tongue coating, deep, thready and weak pulse.

Therapeutic Principles: Warm the kidney and strengthen *yang* for dispersing cold and promoting diuresis.

Recipe: Zhen wu tang

Poria	15 g
Radix Paeoniae Alba	15 g
Rhizoma Atractylodis Macrocephalae	9 g
Radix Aconiti Praeparata	12 g
Rhizoma Zingiberis Recens	3 slices
Herba Asari	3 g
Ramulus Cinnamomi	9 g
Rhizoma Alismatis	9 g

All the above drugs are to be decocted in water for oral administration.

Chinese Patent Medicine

Wu ling san. Take 6 g each time, twice a day.

Acupuncture and Moxibustion

1. Acupuncture: **Fēngchí (GB20)**, **Bǎihuì (DU20)**, **Tàiyáng (EX - HN5)**, **Shàngxīng(DU23)**, **Yìntáng(EX - HN3)**, **Yìfēng(SJ17)**, **Fēnglóng(ST40)**, **Hégǔ(LI4)**, **Tàichōng(LR3)**, **Zúsānlǐ(ST36)**, **Qiángjiān(DU18)** and **Sānyīnjiāo(SP6)**. 3 to 5 points are punctured each time. The treatment is given once every day.

2. Moxibustion: It can be applied on **Zúsānlǐ(ST36)** till local skin becomes hot enough. One moxibustion is given once every day.

Part Four   Commonly Used Recipes

Decoction of Cinnamomi, Glycyrrhizae, etc.
(Guizhi Gancao Longgu Muli Tang)

INGREDIENTS

Ramulus Cinnamomi	10 g
Radix Clycyrrhizae Praeparata	15 g
Os Draconis	30 g
Concha Ostreae	30 g

EFFICACY

Warming heart−yang energy and tranquilizing; mainly for cases attributive to impairment of heart−yang, which manifest palpitation, irritability, spontaneous sweating, pale tongue with white and greasy fur, floating and slow, or slow pulse with irregular intervals.

INDICATIONS

1. For cases attributive to severe deficiency of heart−yang, which manifest sweating, cold limbs, feeble and large or slow and weak pulse, add Radix Aconiti Praeparata to recuperate the depleted yang.

2. Applicable to cases of nocturnal emission with dizziness, fatigue, spiritlessness, reddish tongue, small and slow pulse, which are attributive to ineqilibrium between yin and yang.

3. Also applicable to cases of rheumatic heart disease, sinus bradycardia and atrioventricular block with palpitation, which are attributive to deficiency of heart – yang; and to cases of neurasthenia and hypogonadism with nocturnal emission, which are attributed to inequilibrium of yin and yang.

INTERPRETATION

Glycyrrhizae is used in a large dose in this prescription and serves particulary to relieve palpitation and irritability. In sum, this prescription aims chiefly at warming and promoting heart – yang. Palpitation and other symptoms mentioned above may subside when the heart – yang is restored.

Decoction of Cinnamomi, Paeoniae and Aemarrhenae
(Guizhi Shaoyao Zhimu Tang)

INGREDIENTS

Ramulus Cinnamomi	10 g
Radix Paeoniae Alba	10 g
Rhizoma Zingiberis Recens	10 g
Rhizoma Atractylodis Macrocephalae	10 g
Radix Anemarrhenae	10 g
Radix Ledebouriellae	10 g
Radix Aconiti Praeparata	6 g
Herba Ephedrae	5 g
Radix Glycyrrhizae	3 g

EFFICACY

Expelling wind and dampness, activating yang – energy, relieving arthralgia, regulating yin and clearing away heat, mainly for cases with severe and imgratory arthralgia with swelling and increased temperature of the affected joints, dizzines, fatigue, nausea, vomiting, emaciation, thin and yellow greasy fur on the tongue, rapid pulse, which are attributive to accumulation of wind and dampness with production of heat evil.

INDICATIONS

1. This prescription is suitable for arthralgia of wind – dampness type with formation of heat. It is not indicated for those cases with severe heat which manifest high fever, thirst, red tongue with yellow and dry fur, smooth and rapid bounding pulse.
2. Applicable to cases of apoplexy involving the meridians manifested by hemiplegia, rigidity of limbs, dizziness, thin and yellow greasy fur on the tongue, wiry pulse, which are attributive to prolonged retention of wind and phlegm – dampness in the meridians with transformation of heat.
3. Also applicable to cases of chronic gouty arthritis, rheumatic arthritis, periomarthritis, etc. attributive to accumulation of wind – dampness with trnasformation of heat; and to cases of sequela of cerebrovascular accident and rheumatic cerebrobvasculitis with hemiplegia, which are attributive to retention of wind and phlegm – dampness in the meridians.

INTERPRETATION

Ramulus Cinnamomi, Ledebouriellae, Ephedrae and Atractylodis Macrocephalae are used together to eliminate wind – dampness from both superficies and interior. Paeoniae Alba and Anemarrhenae have the effects of regulating yin and clearing away heat. Aconiti serves to activate yang – energy, expel dampness and alleviate pain when it is used together with Ramulus Cinnamomi, Paeoniae Alba and Anemarrhenae. It is noteworthy that drugs of both hot and cold or yin and yang nature are used simultaneously in the prescription, and their actions are pro-

Commonly Used Recipes

moted each other instead of antagonized.

Antipyretic and Antitoxic Bolus
(Qingwen Jiedu Wan)

Ingredients

Folium Isatidis
Fructus Forsythiae
Radix Scrophulariae
Radix Trichosanthis
Radix Platycodi
Fructus Arctii
Radix Seu Rhizoma Notopterygii
Radix Angelicae Dahuricae
Radix Ledebouriellae
Radix Puerariae
Radix Scutellariae
Radix Bupleuri
Rhizoma Ligustici Chuanxiong
Radix Paeoniae Rubra
Radix Glycyrrhizae
Herba Lophatheri

Efficacy

Having antipyretic and antitoxic functions.
Honey boluses, 9 g each bolus; 10 boluses per box.

Indications

Influenza, marked by fever with chills, anhidrosis with headache, thirst and dry throat, aching pain of limbs. It is also used to treat swelling and pain of mumps.

Administration and Dosage

To be taken orally, one bolus each time, twice a day. For children, the doses should be correspondingly reduced.

Bolus of Calculus Bovis for Purging the Heart – Fire
(Niuhuang qingxin wan)

Ingredients

Calculus Bovis	0.75 g
Cinnabaris	4.5 g
Rhizoma Coptidis	15 g
Radix Scutellariae	9 g
Fructus Gardeniae	9 g
Radix Curcumae	6 g

Indications

Clearing away heat evil and toxic material, waking up patients from unconsciousness by eliminating phlegm; mainly for seasonal febrile diseases with heat evil involving the pericardium and the phlegm – heat evil stagnating in the heart, which are manifested by high fever, irritability, coma, delirium, red tongue with yellowish fur.

Bolus of Citri Grandis
(Juhe wan)

Ingredients

Semen Citri Grandis	30 g
Sargassum	10 g
Thallus Laminariae seu Eckloniae	10 g
Thallus Laminariae Japonicae	10 g
Fructus Meliae Toosendan	10 g
Cortex Magnoliae Officinalis	10 g
Semen Persicae	6 g
Caulis Akebiae	6 g
Radix Aucklandiae	6 g
Lignum Cinnamomi	3 g

Efficacy

Activating circulation of vital qi and blood, dredging the passage of yang – qi, promoting diuresis, dissolving phlegm and softening the hard lumps; mainly for swelling of scrotum due to phlegm – dampness, with pain referred to the abdomen, whitish and greasy fur on the tongue and wiry pulse.

Indications

1. This prescription is applicable to cases with persistent swelling of scrotum. For cases with severe pain, add *Radix Angelicae Sinensis* and *Radix Cyathulae* to eliminate blood stasis and relieving pain; for cases with cold pain, add *Fructus Foeniculi* and *Fructus Evodiae* to warm the liver and expel the cold evil. In cases of transformation to heat from cold – dampness with redness, swelling, itching or yellowish discharge over the scrotum and oliguria, subtract *Lignum Cinnamomi* and add *Cortex Phellodendri*, *Radix Gentianae*, to clear away heat and dampness.

2. For single or multiple, smooth, and painless goiters attributive to stagnation of vital qi and phlegm, subtract *Caulis Akebiae*, and *Meliae Toosendan* and add *Rhizoma Cyperi* and *Bulbus Fritillariae Thunbergii* to promote circulation of vital qi and eliminate phlegm.

3. For cases of breast nodules, unilateral or bilateral, round or oval, smooth or nodular, attributive to stagnation of vital qi and phlegm, subtract *Caulis Akebiae* and add *Fructus hordei Germinatus* (in a large dosage) and *Retinervus Citri Fructus* to disperse the depressed liver − qi and dissolving phlegm.

4. Also applicable to case of hydrocele of tunica vaginalis, varicocele of spermatic cord, thyroid adenoma, breast fibroadenoma, etc. attributive to stagnation of vital qi and phlegm.

Interpretation

Semen Citri Grandis, bitter in taste and warm in nature, is an agent for regulating vital qi, dispersing stagnation and relieving pain. *Meliae Toosendan*, *Aucklandiae*, *Aurantii Immaturus* and *Magnoliae Officinalis* have the effects of dispersing the depressed liver − qi, relieving pain and promoting diuresis. *Laminarriae seu Eckloniae*, *Sargassum* and *Laminariae japonicae* serve to soften hard lumps, dissolve phlegm and disperse stagnation. *Lignum Cinnamomi* together with *Persicae* and *Corydalis* can warm the meridians and activate blood circulation; while together with *Aucklandiae* can promote diuresis and lead the dampness downwards.

Bolus of Rhei and Eupolyphaga seu Steleophaga
(Dahuang zhechong wan)

Ingredients

Radix et Rhizoma Rhei (steamed)	8 g
Eupolyphaga seu Steleophaga	6 g
Radix Scutellariae	6 g
Radix Glycyrrhizae	6 g

Semen Persicae	6 g
Semen Armeniacae Amarum	6 g
Tabanus Bivittatus	6 g
Holotrichia Diomphalia	6 g
Radix Paeoniae Alba	12 g
Radix Rehmanniae	30 g
Dry Lacquer	3 g
Hirudo	8 set

Grind the above ingredients into powder and is prepared as boluses, taken with warm wine.

Efficacy

Eliminating blood stasis and masses, nourishing blood to promote tissue regeneration; mainly for consumptive diseases attributive to retention of blood stasis in the body, which are manifested by emaciation, abdominal fullness, anorexia, squamation and dryness of skin, blackish coloration around the eyes, petechiae on the tongue, wiry and unsmooth pulse, etc..

Indications

1. For cases with localized abdominal pain and tenderness, dry stools, dark purplish tongue, wiry and small, smooth pulse, which are attributive to stagnation of blood and vital energy, hyperactivity of evil and sthenia of healthy energy, the prescription may be used as an analgesic and blood-stasis eliminating agent.

2. Also indicated for cases of erysipelas of the leg with lymphangitis, dark reddish tongue, wiry and unsmooth pulse, which are attributive to obstruction of meridians by blood stasis and heat.

3. Applicable to cases of amenorrhea accompanied with localized aching and marked tenderness over the lower abdomen, emaciation, purplish spots at the margin of the tongue, wiry and small, unsmooth pulse, which are attibutive to the stagnation of liver-blood.

4. Also applicable to cases of cirrhosis of liver, pulmonary tuberculosis, gastric cancer, thrombophlebitis, osteomyelitis, etc., which are attributive to reten-

tion of blood stasis in the body or obstruction of the meridians by blood stasis and heat.

Interpretation

Rhei activates blood circulation and eliminates blood stasis; *Eupolyphaga seu Steleophaga* removes stagnated blood and eliminates masses. They act together to discharge the blood stasis with feces. *Tabanus Bivittatus*, *Holotrichia Diomphalia*, *Lacquer*, *Persicae* and *Hirudo* are applied to activate blood circulation and dredge the passage of meridians, and also applied № 6 to open the stagnated lung – qi and promote blood circulation; they all serve to increase the effect of eliminating blood stasis. № 10, 9 and № 4 can nourish blood and vessels to support healthy energy. № 3 purges stagnancy – heat which may be formed by blood stasis. Wine serves to enhance the effect of other drugs.

Bolus of Six Drugs Including Rehmannia
(Liuwei dihuang wan)

Ingredients

Rhizoma Rehmanniae Praeparata	240 g
Fructus Corni	120 g
Rhizoma Dioscoreae	120 g
Rhizoma Alismatis	90 g
Poria	90 g
Cortex Moutan Radicis	90 g

Grind the drugs into fine powder and mix with honey to make boluses as big as the seed of *Chinese parasol*, to be administered orally 6 – 9 grams each time with warm boiled water or slight salt water, twice or three times a day. The drugs can also be decocted in water for oral administration with the dosage reduced in proportion as the original recipe.

Efficacy

Nourishing and enriching the liver and kidney.

Indications

Syndrome due to the deficiency of vital esence of liver and kidney with symptoms of weakness and soreness of waist and knees, vertigo, tinnitus, deafness, night sweat, emission as well as persistant opening of fontanel. Or the flaring up of sthenic fire resulting in symptoms such as hectic fever, feverish sensation in the palms and soles, diabetes or toothache due to fire of deficiency type, dry mouth and throat, red tongue with little fur, and thready and rapid pusle.

Since it tends to be greasy tonics, the recipe should be administered carefully to patients with weakened function of the spleen in transporting and distributing nutrients and water.

In addition, the above recipe can be modified to treat many other disease indicating the syndrome due to the deficiency of vital essence of liver and kidney such as vegetative nerve functional disturbance, hypertension, arteriosclerosis, diabetes, chronic nephritis, hyperthyroidism, pulmonary tuberculosis, chronic urinary infection, bronchial asthma, amenorrhea, scanty menstruation, or infantile dysplasia and interlectual hypoevolutism.

Interpretation

Prepared *rhizome of rehmannia*, as the principal one, possesses the effect of nourishing the kidney − yin and supplementing the essence of life. As assistant drugs, *dogwood fruit*, sour in flavor and warm in nature, is used for nourishing the kidney and replenishing the liver, while dried **Chinese yam** for nourishing the kidney − yin and tonifying the spleen. The rest ingredients collectively play the role of adjuvant drus. **Oriental water plantain** coordinates with the principal drug in clearing the kidney and purging turbid evils, *moutan bark* cooperates with dogwood fruit in purging liver fire, and poria shares the effort together with dried *Chinese yam* to excrete dampness from the spleen. The whole recipe acts as both tonics and purgatives with tonifying effect dominant.

Clinically and experimentally, the recipe has the effects of nourishing the body and consolidating the constitution, inhibiting hypercatabolism, reducing excitement of the brain, adjusting endocrine function and vegetative nerve, lowering blood pressure and blood sugar, inducing diuresis, improving the function of the kidney as well as promoting the epithelial hyperplasia of the esophagus and preventing cancer, etc..

Bolus of Ten Powerful Tonics
(Shiquan dabu wan)

Ingredients

Radix Codonopsis Pilosulae
Rhizoma Atractylodis Macrocephalae
Poria
Radix Glycyrrhizae
Radix Angelicae Sinensis
Rhizoma Ligustici Chuanxiong
Radix Paeoniae Alba
Radix Rehmanniae Praeparata
Radix Astragali seu Hedysari
Cortex Cinnamomi

Honeyed boluses, 9 g each bolus, 10 boluses per box. To be taken orally, one bolus each time, twice or three times daily.

Efficacy

Warming and nourishing qi and blood.

Indications

Deficiency of both qi and blood marked by sallow complexion, short breath, palpitation, dizziness, spontaneous perspiration, mental fatigue, lassitude of the extremities, profuse menstruation. It also serves as a supporting drug to detoxicating drugs in the treatment of non-healing of ulcers due to deficiency of qi and blood.

Cow-bezoar Bolus for Clearing Away Heat of the Upper Part of the Body
(Niuhuang shang qing wan)

Ingredients

Calculus Bovis
Herba Menthae
Flos Schizonepetae
Radix Ligustici Chuanxiong
Fructus Gardeniae
Rhizoma Coptidis
Cortex Phellodendri
Radix Scutellariae
Radix et Rhizoma Rhei
Fructus Forsythiae
Radix Paeoniae Rubra
Radix Angelicae Sinensis
Radix Rehmanniae
Radix Platycodi
Gypsum Fibrosum
Borneolum
Radix Glycyrrhizae

Grind the above drugs into fine powder, mix it with honey and make them into boluses, 6 g each bolus, 10 boluses per box.

Administration and Dosage

To be taken orally, one bolus each time, twice a day.

Efficacy

Clearing away heat and purging pathogenic fire, dispelling wind and relieving pain.

Commonly Used Recipes

Indications

The syndromes of excessive fire in the middle and upper parts of the human body or the attack of pathogenic wind and heat on the upper part of the body marked by headache, vertigo, conjunctival congestion, tinnitus, swelling and sore throat, ulcerations of the mouth and tongue, swelling and soreness of the gums, constipation and dry stool.

Cautions

Pregnant women should be careful when taking this medicine.

Decoction for Clearing Away Pestilent Factors and Detoxification
(Qingwen baidu yin)

Ingredients

Cornu Rhinocerotis	18 – 24 g; 9 – 15 g; 6 – 12 g
Rhizoma Coptidis	12 – 18 g; 6 – 12 g; 3 – 5 g
Fructus Gardeniae	6 – 9 g
Radix Platycodi	6 – 9 g
Radix Scutellariae	6 – 9 g
Rhizoma Anemarrhenae	6 – 9 g
Radix Paeoniae Rubra	6 – 9 g
Radix Scrophulariae	6 – 9 g
Fructus Forsythiae	6 – 9 g
Radix Glycyrrhizae	6 – 9 g
Cortex Moutan Radicis	6 – 9 g
Herba Lophatheri	6 – 9 g

Efficacy

Clearing away heat evil and toxic materials, cooling blood and supporting yin; mainly fro cases of seasonal epidemic diseses attributive to hyperactivity of severe heat in qifen and xuefen, which are manifested by high fever, restlessness, or even mania and delirium, thirst, intense headache, purplish red eruptions, hematemesis, epistaxis, dry lips, crimson tongue, rapid pulse.

Indications

1. The prescription is widely applicable to cases of internal medicine and surgery.

2. For critical cases of furunculosis complicated by septicemia attributive to the attack of viscera by toxic material, add *Flos Lonicerae* and omit *Lophatheri* and *Scrophulariae*.

3. For cases with general aching, intense headache, lumbago, oliguria, high fever, irritability, which are attributive to the attack of fire and pestilent evil, omit *Platycodi* and *Glycyrrhizae* and add *Rhizoma Imperatae* to nourish yin and promote diuresis. Nowadays, it is also applied for cases of leptosprosis with the above symptoms.

4. For cases with discharge of fresh or darkish bloody stools, high fever, irritability, red tongue, dry lips, sunken and small, rapid pulse, which are attributive to severe attack of pestilent evil, omit *Glycyrrhizae*, *Platycodi*, *Lophatheri*, *Forsythiae* and add *Flos Carthami*. Nowadays, it is also applied for cases of necrotizing enterocolitis with the same mechanism.

5. Also applicable to epidmeic meningitis, scarlet fever, erysipelas of face, septicemia, etc. attributive to the attack of pestilent evil and hyperactivity of heat in qifen and xuefen.

Interpretation

This prescription is composed of the modificatins of *White tiger decoction*, *Decoction of Coptidis for Detoxification* and *Decoction of Cornu Rhioncerotis and Rehmanniae*. *Gypsum Fibrosum*, *Anemarrhenae*, *Glycyrrhizae* and

Lophatheri have the effect of clearing away sthenic heat in qifen. *Coptidis*, *Gardeniae*, *Scutellariae* and *Forsythiae* have the effects of puring fire and elimination toxic materials. *Cornu Rhinocerotis*, *Rehmanniae*, *Moutan Radicis*, *Paeoniae Rubra* and *Scrophulariae* have the effects of cooling blood and preserving ying. The combination of three prescriptions constituents a strong agent for clearing away heat evil and toxic material.

Decoction for Clearing Heat in Ying System
(Qing ying tang)

Ingredients

Cornu Rhinocerotis	2 g
Radix Rehmanniae	15 g
Radix Scrophulariae	9 g
Herba Lophatheri	3 g
Radix Ophiopogonis	9 g
Radix Salviae Miltiorrhizae	6 g
Rhizoma Coptidis	5 g
Flos Lonicerae	9 g
Fructus Forsythiae	6 g

All the above drugs are to be decocted in water for oral administration.

Efficacy

Clearing and dispelling pathogenic heat from ying system, nourishing yin and promoting blood circulation.

Indications

Invasion of ying system by pathogenic heat manifested by feverish body which is aggravated in the night, delirium, insomnia due to vexation, or by faint skin rashes, deep-red and dry tongue and rapid pulse.

The recipe can also be modified to deal with ying-syndrome occuring in epidemic encephalitis B, epidemic cerebrospinal meningitis, septicemia and other infectious diseases.

Interpretation

In the recipe, *Cornu Rhinocerotis*, being salty in flavour and cold in property, and *Radix Rehmanniae* being sweet in taste and cold in nature, both exert a role of a principal drug, having the effect of removing heat from ying and blood systems. *Scrophulariae* and *Ophiopogonis* together act as assistant drugs having the effect of nourishing yin and clearing heat. The rest share the role of adjuvant and guiding drugs. *Lophatheri*, *Ophiopogonis*, *Lonicerae* and *Forsythiae* are used to clear and dispel pathogenic heat from ying system through qi system, and *Salviae Miltiorrhizae* is used to promote blood circulation to remove blood stasis.

Clinically and Experimentally, it is ascertained that the recipe possesses the efficacies of relieving inflammation, bringing down fever, tranquilizing the mind, resisting bacteria and viruses, tonifying the heart, arresting bleeding improving immunologic function, promoting blood circulation and so on.

Cases with white and slippery coating of the tongue which suggests invasion by pathogenic dampness should not use recipe in case it encourages pathogenic dampness.

Decoction for Strngthening Middle Jiao and Benefiting Vital Energy
(Bu zhong yi qi tang)

Ingredients

Radix Astragali seu Hedysari	15 g
Radix Codonopsis Pilosulae	15 g
Radix Angelicae Sinensis	10 g
Rhizoma Atractylodis Macrodephalae	10 g
Exocarpium Citri Grandis	6 g
Radix Glycyrrhizae Praeparata	6 g

Rhizoma Cimicifugae	3 g
Radix Bupleuri	3 g
Fructus Ziziphi Jujubae	6 g
Rhizoma Zingiberis Recens	6 g

Decoct the above ingredients in a right amount of water for oral administration.

Efficacy

Strengthening spleen, benefiting qi, lifting up yang – qi, mainly for the cases with deficiency of spleen and stomach and collapse of middle – jiao energy, manifested by shortness of breath, disinclination for speaking, tiredness, weakness, or prolapse of rectum, or fever due to deficiency of qi, pale tongue with white fur, empty and weak pulse.

Indications

1. This prescription is originally applied to fever due to internal damage, and now commonly for prolapse of rectum, gastroptosis and prolapse of uterus due to deficiency and collapse of qi.

2. Applicable to cases of common cold with deficiency of qi manifesting lingering fever, profuse sweating, pale tongue and weak pulse.

3. Also applicable to cases of septicemia, pulmonary tuberculosis, aplastic anemia, leukemia and summer fever which are manifested by fever due to deficiency of qi.

Interpretation

Astragali seu Hedysari has the effects of tonifying and lifting up qi; № 2, 4 and № 6 have the effects of strengthening the spleen and regulating the stomach, helping № 1 to tonify qi. While № 7 and № 8 have the effects of leading the stomach – qi upward, helping № 1 to lift up qi. № 3 can nourish blood and help qi to flow toward its bases. The case with deficiency of qi usually suffers from stagnation of qi, so the prescription includes № 5, 10 and № 9 to regulate qi and the stomach.

Modern studies have confirmed that the recipe has the efficacies in improving the cellular immune function promoting metabolism, improving the excitement of cerebral cortex, promoting the tension of skeletal muscles, smooth muscles and supporting tissues; and promoting digestion and absorption.

Cautions

Patients with internal heat due to yin deficiency is prohibited from taking this recipe, and for those with the impairment of body fluid and qi after illness, it's better to prescribe this recipe together with other drugs.

Decoction of Arctii for Soothing Muscles
(Niubang jieji tang)

Ingredients

Fructus Arctii	12 g
Fructus Forsythiae	12 g
Radix Scrophulariae	12 g
Fructus Gardeniae	10 g
Cortex Moutan Radicis	10 g
Spica Prunellae	10 g
Herba Dendrobii	10 g
Herba Schizonepetae	6 g
Herba Menthae	3 g

Decoct the above ingredients in a right amount of water for oral administration.

Efficacy

Clearing away heat and toxic material, expelling wind from the body surface and reducing swelling; mainly for skin infection of the head and neck, accompanied with fever, chilliness, headache, dry mouth, oliguria with reddish urine, red tongue with yellow fur, smooth and rapid pulse, which are attributive to the attack of wind, fire, toxic material and heat.

Indications

1. Applicable to cases of common cold attributive to attack of exogenous wind – heat, which manifest as fever, chilliness, headache, sore – throat, thirst, thinyellow fur on the tongue, floating and rapid pulse.

2. For cases of measles with interrupted eruption, fever, chilliness, sneezing, cough, congestion of conjunctiva, lacrimation, thirst, red tongue with thin yellow fur, floating and rapid pulse, which are attributive to attack of heat and toxic material to the lung and stomach, and retention of the pathogens in the superficies.

3. Also to cases of hordeolum accompanied with fever, chilliness, headache, thirst, red tongue and rapid pulse, which are attributive to attack of heat and toxic material to the eyes.

4. For cases of upper respiratory viral infection and inffluenza attributive to the attack of exogenous wind – heat; and for cases of chalazion and tarsitis attributive to the attack of heat evil and toxic material attack to the eyes.

Interpretation

Arctii acts as the principal drug of the prescription, which can expel wind and heat, eliminate toxic material and relieve swelling. *Schizonepetae*, *Menthae* help *Arctii* to disperse wind – heat from the head and face. *Forsythiae*, *Prunellae*, *Moutan Radicis*, *Gardeniae* and *Scrophulariae* , when used together with *Schizonepetae* and *Menthae*, serve to eliminate heat and toxic material from the head and face, to expel wind from the body surface and to relieve swelling. Because the retention of heat and toxic material can damage the yin – fluid, *Dendrobii* is applied to nourish yin and promote the production of body fluid. When the body fluid is sufficient, the high body temperature may become normal.

Decoction of Coptidis for Detoxification
(Neishu huanglian tang)

Ingredients

Rhizoma Coptidis	9 g
Radix Scutellariae	9 g
Fructus Gardeniae	9 g
Fructus Forsythiae	9 g
Radix Angelicae Sinensis	9 g
Radix Paeoniae Alba	9 g
Radix Aucklandiae	6 g
Herba Menthae	3 g
Radix Platycodi	3 g
Radix Glycyrrhizae	3 g
Radix et Rhizoma Rhei	6 g

Decoct the above ingredients in a right amount of water for oral administration.

Efficacy

Clearing away heat and toxic material, activating blood circulation, relieving swelling and promoting bowel movement.

Indications

To cases of jaundice manifested by bright yellow coloration over the body, fever, thirst, oliguria, reddish urine, constipation, yellow and greasy fur on the tongue, wiry and rapid pulse, which are attributive to the accumulation of dampness-heat.

To cases of appendicitis, liver abscess and lung abscess, to cases of cellulitis, lymphadenitis and mastitis and to cases of acute cholecystitis, icterus infectious hepatitis and cholelithiasis with jaundice attributive to the attack of dampness-heat.

Interpretation

Coptidis, *Scutellariae* and *Gardeniae* have the effects of clearing away heat evil and toxic material from the interior. *Menthae*, *Forsythiae* and *Platycodi* enhance the effects of the above drugs. *Angelicae Sinensis*, *Paeoniae Alba* and *Aucklandiae* serve to promote the circulation of vital qi and blood, and relieve swelling and pain. *Arecae* and *Rhei* promote the circulation of vital qi and bowel movement to purge the fire from below. *Glycyrrhizae* serves to increase the effect of *Rhei*. In sum, this prescription is designed for eliminating heat and toxic material both from the interior and the superficies.

Decoction of Cinnamomi Adding Cinnamomi
(Guizhi jia gui tang)

Ingredients

Ramulus Cinnamomi	15 g
Radix Paeoniae Alba	10 g
Rhizoma Zingiberis Recens	10 g
Radix Glycyrrhizae Praeparata	6 g
Fructus Ziziphi Jujubae	8 pcs

Decoct the above ingredients in a right amount of water for oral administration.

Efficacy

Activating yang – energy, eliminating cold, lowering adverse rising qi; mainly for cases attributive to attack of exogenous cold and adverse rising of cold originally retained in the lower jiao, which manifest feeling of an air flow moving from the lower abdomen upward to the chest and throat, abdominal pain, vomiting, intolerance of cold, white and greasy fur on the tongue, wiry and tense pulse.

Indications

Applicable to cases attributive to accumulation of yin − cold in the collaterals of jueyin, which manifest induration, swelling and pain of the scrotum, preference for warmth and aversion to cold, cold feet, white and greasy fur on the tongue, sunken and wiry pulse.

For cases with palpitation, frightening, feeling of fullness over the chest, cold limbs, white and greasy fur on the tongue, which are attributive to hypofunction of heart − yang, increase the dosage of *Glycyrrhizae Praeparata*.

Also applicable to cases of spasmodic colon and gastro − intestinal neurosis attributive to adverse rising of interior cold accompanied with the attack of exogenous cold; to cases of indirect inguinal hernia and inguinal hernia attributive to the accumulation of yin − cold; and also to cases of sinus arrhythmia and atrioventricular block attributive to hypofunction of heart − yang.

Interpretation

This prescription is composed by adding an extra dose of *Ramulus Cinnamomi* or *Cortex Cinnamomi* to the *Decoction of Ramulus Cinnamomi*. *Ramulus Cinnamomi* is used to disperse cold from the superficies and to lower the adverse rising qi, and serves as the principal drug of the prescription for both symptomatic and causative treatment. *Paeoniae Alba* serves to regulate ying and wei and to promote diaphoresis when it is used together with *Ramulus Cinnamomi*. It can also relieve pain and prevent abnormal rising of liver − qi when it is used together with *Glycyrrhizae Praeparata*. *Zingiberis Recens* can clear away cold, promote sweating and lower the adverse rising qi when it combines with *Ramulus Cinnamomi*, and can regulate ying and wei and warm the spleen and stomach when it combines with *Ziziphi Jujubae*. *Glycyrrhizae Praeparata* used with *Ramulus Cinnamomi* can relieve abnormal throbbing.

Decoction for General Antiphlogistic
(Puji xiaodu yin)

Ingredients

Radix Scutellariae	15 g
Rhizoma Coptidis	15 g
Fructus Forsythiae	10 g
Radix Isatidis	10 g
Radix Scrophulariae	10 g
Fructus Arctii	10 g
Exocarpium Citri Grandis	6 g
Radix Glycyrrhizae	6 g
Radix Bupleuri	6 g
Radix Platycodi	6 g
Lasiosphaera seu Calvatia	3 g
Herba Menthae	3 g
Bombyx Batryticatus	3 g
Rhizoma Cimicifugae	3 g

Decoct the above ingredients in a right amount of water for oral administration.

Efficacy

Clearing away heat evil and toxic material, expelling wind evil from the body surface, relieving swelling; mainly for some epidemic diseases attributive to the accumulation of wind, heat and pestilent evil in the head and face, manifested by swelling, redness and pain over the face, chilliness, fever, sore-throat, reddish tongue with white and yellow fur, floating and rapid, strong pulse, etc..

Indications

1. This is a representative prescription for treating the epidemic diseases characterized by swelling and redness of face. When the superficies-syndrome

has subsided and heat-syndrome becomes prominent. *Menthae* and *Bupleuri* should be subtracted and *Flos Lonicerae* added.

2. Applicable to furunculosis of the face and head attributive to upward attack of heat evil and toxic material (usually add *Lonicerae* and *Herba Schizonepetae*, and subtract *Lasiosphaera seu Calvatia* and *Bupleuri*).

3. Also applicable to cases of acute tonsillitis, acute otitis media, acute lymphadentis, mumps, etc., attributive to accumulation of wind-heat and pestilent evil in the head. In cases of mumps complicated by orchitis, add *Fructus Meliae Toosendan* to purge the sthenic fire of liver meridian.

Interpretation

Scutellariae and *Coptidis* are used in large dose to clear away heat evil and toxic material from the upper jiao. *Forsythiae*, *Arctii*, *Bombyx Batryticatus* and *Menthae* serve to expel wind-heat evil from the upper jiao. *Scrophulariae* and *Isatidis* enhance the effects of *Scutellariae*, and *Coptidis*, *Lasiosphaera seu Calvatia*, *Platycodi* and *Glycyrrhizae* are assisted by *Arctii* and *Menthae* to ease the throat. *Exocarpium Citri Grandis* has the effects of regulating vital energy and helps above drugs to expel wind evil and relieve swelling. *Cimicifugae* and *Bupleuri* can expel wind-heat evil and helps the above drugs distributing to the head and face. This is a well-known prescription for clearing away heat evil and toxic material.

Decoction for Purging Liver-fire and Eliminating Dampness (Qing gan sheng shi tang)

Ingredients

Radix Scutellariae	10 g
Fructus Gardeniae	10 g
Radix Angelicae Sinensis	10 g
Radix Paeoniae Alba	10 g
Radix Trichosanthis	10 g

Radix Rehmanniae	20 g
Rhizoma Ligustici Chuanxiong	6 g
Radix Bupleuri	6 g
Radix Gentianae	6 g
Rhizoma Alismatis	6 g
Caulis Akebiae	6 g
Medulla Junci	3 g
Radix Glycyrrhizae	3 g

Decoct the above ingredients in a right amount of water for oral administration.

Efficacy

Clearing away heat and dampness, dispersing the stagnated liver – qi, alleviating pain, activating the circulation of blood and relieving swelling; mainly for cases of scrotitis with chilliness, fever, oliguria, red tongue with yellow and greasy fur, wiry and rapid pulse, which are attributive to downward attack of dampness – heat from the liver meridian and the stagnation of blood and toxic materials.

Indications

1. For cases with induration, pain and swelling of testis, erythema and hotness of the scrotum, accompanied with chilliness, fever, headache, thirst, oliguria with deep – colored urine, red tongue with yellow and greasy fur, wiry and rapid pulse, which are attributive to downward attack of dampness – heat to the collateral of "jueyin" and the stagnation of blood and toxic material, add *Fructus Meliae Toosendan*, or *Semen Citri Grandis*, and omit *Glycyrrhizae* and *Junci*.

2. Also applicable to cases of hydrocele of tunica vaginalis, varicocele of spermatic cord, orchitis, tuberculosis of testis, etc. attributive to downward attack of dampness – heat and stagnation of blood and toxic material.

Interpretation

This prescription is formed by adding *Ligustici Chuanxiong*, *Paeoniae Alba*, *Trichosanthis* and *Junci*, and omitting *Semen Plantaginis* from the *Decoction of Gentianae for purging liver – fire*. In this prescription, *Gardeniae*, *Scutellariae* and *Gentianae* serve to purge the heat – toxic material from the liver meridian, and *Akebiae*, *Junci* and *Alismatis* to eliminate the dampness – toxic material from the lower – jiao. *Angelicae Sinensis*, *Rehmanniae*, *Paeoniae Alba*, *Ligustici Chuanxiong* are used together with *Bupleuri* to activate blood circulation, relieve swelling, disperse the stagnated liver – qi and alleviate pain. *Trichosanthis* has the effects of clearing away heat and eliminating phlegm, and promotes the subsidence of swelling. *Glycyrrhizae* serves to clear away heat and toxic material.

Golden Lock Bolus for Keep Kidney Essence
(Jinsuo gu jing wan)

Ingredients

Semen Astragali Complanati	30 g
Semen Euryales	30 g
Semen Nelumbinis	30 g
Stamen Nelumbinis	15 g
Os Draconis	20 g
Concha Ostreae	20 g

Efficacy

Strengthening kidney essence and stopping nocturnal emission; mainly for cases with hypofunction of kidney, characterized by nocturnal emission, fatigue, sorenss of limbs, lumbago, tinnitus, pale tongue with whitish fur, small and weak pulse.

Indications

1. Applicable to deficiency of both kidney-yin and yang. For cases with deficiency of kidney-yin predominantly, add Fructus Ligustri Lucidi and Fructus Rosae Laevigatae, while for those with deficiency of kidney-yang predominantly, add Fructus Psoraleae and Pulvis of Cornu Cervi. It is not suitabld for nocturnal emission due to hyperactivity of "prime-minister" fire.

2. For cases of leukorrhagia with thin discharge, attributive to deficiency of spleen-yang and yin, omit Stamen Nelumbinis and add Poria and Rhizoma Atractylodis Macrocephalae (in large dosage) to invigorate the spleen and kidney).

3. Applicable to cases of neurasthenia with nocturnal emission, and cervicitis with leukorrhagia, which are attributive to hypofunction of kidney.

Interpretation

Complanati has the effects of invigorating kidney, supporting kidney essence and stopping nocturnal emission. *Semen Nelumbinis* and *Semen Euryales* serve to clear away heart-fire, benefit the kidney and keep heart-fire and kidney-water in balance. *Os Draconis*, *Concha Ostreae* and *Stamen Nelumbinis* can relieve nocturnal emission and calm the mental state. All the above drugs constituent a prescription effective for arresting nocturnal emission.

Zaizao Powder
(Zaizao san)

Ingredients

Radix Astragali seu Hedysari	12 g
Radix codonopsis Pilosulae	10 g
Ramulus Cinnamomi	6 g
Radix Paeoniae Alba	6 g
Radix Aconiti Praeparata	6 g
Rhizoma seu Radix Notopterygii	6 g

Radix Ledebouriellae	6 g
Rhizoma Ligustici Chuanxiong	6 g
Herba Asari	3 g
Radix Glycyrrhizae Praeparata	3 g
Rhizoma Zingiberis Recens	5 pcs
Fructus Ziziphi Jujubae	2 pcs0

Efficacy

Supporting yang — qi to promote sweating, benefiting vital qi and expelling superficial evils from body surface; mainly for cases of common cold of wind — cold type with a yang — deficiency constitution, manifested by fever with predominant chilliness, headache, rigidity of neck, anhidrosis, cold limbs, tiredness, pale complexion, low voice, pale tongue with whitish fur, sunken and weak pulse or floating and large, weak pulse, etc..

Indications

1. Applicable to the early stage of pyogenic infection of skin, manifested by local swelling and pain but no erythema nor heat, with predominant fever, chilliness, anhidrosis, cold limbs, no thirst, thin and whitish fur on the tongue, floating and large, weak pulse, which are attributive to attack of exogenous wind — cold and deficiency of yang — qi in the body.
2. Also indicated for cases of arthralgia with wandering pain, chilliness, fever, anhidrosis, cold limbs, tiredness, flat taste of the mouth, floating and large, weak pulse, which are attributive to attack of wind — cold — dampness evil to a person with yang — deficiency constitution.
3. Also applicable to cases of upper respiratory infection, mumps, rheumatic fever, rheumatoid arthritis, carbuncle, furuncle, acute cellulitis, etc., marked by chilliness and fever, which are attributive to deficiency of yang — qi and the attack of exogenous wind — cold — dampness or wind — cold evil.

Interpretation

This prescription is characterized by simultaneous application of cold-expelling and yang-supporting drugs. *Ramulus cinnamomi*, *Notopterygii*, *Ledebouriellae*, *Asari*, *Ligustici Chuanxiong* and *Zingiberis Recens* are diaphoretics for expelling cold. If only diaphoretics are used for those cases with a yang-deficiency constitution, not only perspiration does not occur but also the deficiency of yang would be aggravated, or even yang exhaustion after profuse sweating may ensue. So *Astragali seu Hedysari* and *Codonopsis* are applied to benefit yang-qi, and *Aconiti* is helpful for strengthen yang and promoting sweating. *Paeoniae Alba* and *Ziziphi Jujubae* can nourish blood. When used together with *Astragali seu Hedysari*, *Paeoniae Alba* exerts an astringent effect to prevent over sweating.

Powder for Antiphlogosis
(Baidu san)

Ingredients

Rhizoma seu Radix Notopterygii	12 g
Radix Angelicae Pubescentis	12 g
Radix Bupleuri	10 g
Radix Peucedani	10 g
Rhizoma Ligustici Chuanxiong	10 g
Radix Codonopsis Pilosulae	6 g
Fructus Aurantii	6 g
Poria	6 g
Radix Platycodi	6 g
Radix Glycyrrhizae	3 g
Herba Menthae	3 g
Rhizoma Zingiberis Recens	3 pcs

Decoct the above ingredients in a right amount of water for oral administration.

Efficacy

Benefiting vital qi and expelling the evils from the body surface, eliminating the wind and dampness evil; mainly for cases with insufficiency of healthy qi and attacked by exogenous wind, cold and dampness evil, which are manifested by chilliness, fever, headache, no sweating, general aching, stuffy nose, heavy voice, productive cough, whitish and greasy fur on the tongue, floating and weak pulse, etc..

Indications

1. Applicable to skin infections which are attributive to wind – cold – dampness superficies – syndrome.
2. By adding *Fructus Forsythiae* and *Flos Lonicerae*, and omitting *Codonopsis Pilosulae*, another prescription named *Powder of Forsythiae for Antiphlogosis* is formed. It is indicated for the initial stage of skin infections attributive to virulent heat evil attacking the superficies.
3. By adding *Herba Schizonepetae* and *Radix Ledebouriellae* and omitting *Codonopsis Pilosulae*, *Zingiberis Recens* and *Menthae*, another prescription named *Powder of Schizonepetae and Ledebouriellae for Antiphlogosis* is formed. It is indicated for affections of exogenous wind, cold and dampness evil, which are manifested by chilliness, fever, heavy sensation of head and body, cough, heavy voice, white and greasy fur on the tongue, wiry and tense pulse, etc..
4. Also applicable to cases of influenza, emphysema complicated by infection, malaria, acute cellulitis, etc., which are attirbutive to the affection of wind, cold and dampness evil in cases of the insufficiency of healthy qi.

Interpretation

Notopterygii and *Angelicae Pubescentis* not only can disperse wind – cold evil, but also can eliminate dampness and relieve pain. The former distributes upwardly and the latter downwardly, and they act on the whole body when used together. A small amount of *Codonopsis Pilosulae* is applied together with *Bupleuri*, *Ligustici Chuanxiong*, *Zingiberis Recens* and *Menthae* to invigorate vital qi and expel the evil factors from the body surface by sweating. A small amount of *Poria* is applied together with those drugs of *Peucedani*, *Aurantii* and *Platycodi* to eliminate sputum and relieve cough. *Radix Glycyrrhizae* serves to regulate the other drugs. This prescription combines both tonics and diaphoretics together, and possesses the advantage of producing sweating but not damaging the healthy qi, and that of supporting the healthy qi but not retaining the evils.

Pill of Six Miraculous Drugs
(Liushen wan)

Ingredients

Margarita	4.5 g
Calculus Bovis	4.5 g
Moschus	4.5 g
Realgar	3 g
Borneolum Syntheticum	3 g
Venenum Bufonis	3 g

Coated with burnt herbal powder.

Efficacy

Clearing away heat and toxic material, relieving swelling and alleviating pain; mainly for cases of scarlet fever and tonsillitis with red tongue and rapid pulse, which are attributive to the accumulation of phlegm, fire and toxic material.

Indications

1. The prescription cannot be applied as a decoction for oral use. Some ingredients such as *Realgar* and *Venenum Bufonis* are poisonous, so it should not be taken in alrge dose nor for a long period and is contraindicated for pregnant women.

2. Applicable to carbuncle, furuncle, abscess of breast, and various local infection of unknown origin, which are attributive to accumulation of phlegm, fire and toxic material.

3. Also applicable to cases of pharyngitis, follicular stomatitis, mastitis, nasopharyngeal carcinoma, lung cancer, etc. which are attributive to accumulation of phlegm, fire and toxic material.

The recipe can be modified to deal with influenza, epidemic encephalitis B, epidemic cerebrospinal meningitis, pneumonia and septicemia indicating excessive heat syndrome in the qi system, and also with the treatment of stomatitis, periodontitis, gastritis, diabetes and others which pertain to stomach heat syndrome.

Interpretation

Calculus Bovis, *Realgar* and *Venenum Bufonis* are principal drugs in the prescrription, which have strong and fast effect of eliminating toxic materials and dispersing the accumulation of evils. *Calculus Bovis* can eliminate heat – phlegm, *Realgar* can disperse the stagnated substance, and *Venenum Bufonis* can relieve swelling and alleviate pain. They all are potent agents for clearing away heat and dispelling toxic material, and serve as the principal drugs of the prescription. *Margarita* can clear away heart – fire and eliminate phlegm when it combines with *Calculus Bovis*. *Borneolum Syntheticum* can disperse heat and alleviate pain, and also increase the effect of the other drugs with it combining with *Moschus*. *Burnt herbal powder* has the effect of dispersing the stagnated substance and easing the throat, and is especially good for the infection of oral cavity. In sum, the prescription has a strong detoxifying and swelling – subsiding effect by utilizing the fragrant nature of the ingredients.

Cautions

It is not advisable for those whose exterior syndrome is not relieved, nor for those who have fever due to blood – deficiency or cold syndrome with pseudo – heat symptoms.

Decoction of Phragmitis
(Weijing tang)

Ingredients

Rhizoma Phragmitis	60 g
Semen Coicis	30 g
Semen Benincasae	30 g
Semen Persicae	10 g

Decoct the above ingredients in a right amount of water for oral administration.

Efficacy

Clearing away lung-heat and eliminating sputum, removing blood stasis and pus; mainly for cases of pulmonary abscess with expectoration of foul, purulent and bloody sputum, chest pain aggravated by coughing, red tongue with yellow, greasy fur, smooth and rapid pulse.

Indications

1. This is a typical prescription for pulmonary abscess. For cases without formation of pus, add *Radix Platycodi* and *Bulbus Fritillariae Cirrhosae* to enhance the effect of eliminating the sputum and the pus.

2. For cases of measles after the occurrence of skin eruptions, but still with fever, productive cough, red tongue with yellow greasy fur, smooth and rapid pulse, which are attributive to lung-heat, omit *Persicae* and add *Cortex Mori Radicis* and *Bulbus Fritillariae Thunbergii*.

3. *Also applicable to cases of lobar pneumonia, bronchitis, whooping cough, etc. which are attributive to lung-heat.*

Interpretation

Phragmitis has the effects of clearing away lung-heat and is the principal remedy for pulmonary abscess. *Benincasae* eliminates sputum and pus. *Coicis* clears away heat-evil and promotes diuresis. *Persciae* removes blood stasis and pus. All of these three seeds can also move the bowels and eliminate the pus and blood stasis through defecation. These constitute and ideal prescription for pulmonary abscess of sputum-heat pattern or sputum-blood-stasis pattern. The abscess can be dispersed when the pus is not yet formed, and the pus can be eliminated when the abscess is formed.

Powder of Lonicerae and Forsythiae
(Yinqiao san)

Ingredients

Flos Lonicerae	12 g
Fructus Forsythiae	12 g
Fructus Arctii	10 g
Semen Sojae Praeparatum	10 g
Rhizoma Phragmitis	10 g
Radix Platycodi	5 g
Herba Menthae	5 g
Herba Lophatheri	5 g
Radix Glycyrrhizae	5 g
Spica Schizonepetae	5 g

Efficacy

Expelling wind and heat evil, clearing away heat evil and toxic material; mainly for cases due to exogenous wind and heat evil, which are manifested by fever, mild chilliness, sore-throat, headache, thirst, red tip of the tongue with thin white fur or thin yellowish fur, floating and rapid pulse, etc..

Indications

1. The therapeutic principle of this prescription is reasonable, the concept of compatibility is strict and its curative effect is fruitful, and has become a typical recipe for common cold of wind − heat type. For cases with extreme thirst, add *Radix Trichosanthis* to promote the production of saliva and quench thirst; for cases with sore − throat, add *Radix Scrophulariae* to clear away the heat evil and ease the throat.

2. For the initial stage of measles attributive to stagnation of wind and heat evil in the superficies, which is manifested by fever, thirst and incomplete eruption, add *Radix Puerariae* to let out the eruptions.

3. For cases at the onset of skin infections attributive to super ficies − syndrome of wind − heat type, add *Herba Taraxaci* or *Folium Isatidis* to clear away heat evil and toxic material, and dispersing the accumulation of evils.

4. Also applicable to cases of acute tonsillitis, influenza, mumps, measles, encephalitis $_B$ epidemic meningitis and acute suppurative infection, which are attributive to wind − heat syndrome of the superficies.

Interpretation

Lonicerae and *Forsythiae* are selected as principal drugs which have mild action to let the evil out of the body and clear away heat evil and toxic material, so as to prevent the evil from attacking the interior. *Schizonepetae*, *Menthae* and *Sojae Praeparatum* can expel the evils from the surface of the body owing to their acrid flavour. *Arctii*, *Platycodi* and *Glycyrrhizae* have the effects of clearing away heat evil and toxic material to ease the throat. *Lophatheri* and *Phragmitis* have the effects of clearing away heat evil and promoting the production of body fluid to relieve thirst. This prescription constitutes an acrid − cool remedy by combining the drugs of clearing away heat evil and toxic material with those of expelling the evil from the body surface. This model of compatibility exerts a great influence upon the later generation, and many new set prescriptions for common cold are composed of its modifications.

Powder of Ledebouriellae for Dispersing the Superficies
(Fangfeng tongsheng san)

Ingredients

Radix Ledebouriellae	10 g
Fructus Forsythiae	10 g
Fructus Gardeniae	10 g
Herba Schizonepetae	6 g
Herba Ephedrae	6 g
Rhizoma Ligustici Chuanxiong	6 g
Radix Angelicae Sinensis	6 g
Radix Paeoniae Alba	6 g
Rhizoma Atractylodis Macrocephalae	6 g
Radix et Rhizoma Rhei	6 g
Natrii Sulfas	6 g
Radix Scutellariae	6 g
Talcum	20 g
Gypsum Fibrosum	15 g
Herba Menthae	3 g
Radix Platycodi	3 g
Radix Glycyrrhizae	3 g
Rhizoma Zingiberis Recens	3 pcs

Decoct the above ingredients in a right amount of water for oral administration.

Efficacy

Expelling wind from the body surface, clearing away heat and promoting bowel movement; mainly for sthenia − syndrome of both the superficies and the interior after the attack of exogenous wind − heat and the retention of heat in the interior, which is manifested by aversion to cold, fever, dizziness, bitter and dry mouth, conjunctivitis, sore − throat, feeling of oppression over the chest, constipation, dysuria with reddish urine, red tongue with white or yellow fur, floating and smooth, rapid pulse.

Indications

1. Applicable to cases of early stage of superficial pyogenic infection with local signs of inflammation, chilliness, fever, bitter mouth, constipation, oliguria, red tongue with white fur, floating and rapid pulse.

2. Also indicated for cases of urticaria and eczema with thin and white fur on the tongue, floating and rapid pulse, which are attributive to simultaneous existence of sthenia – syndrome in the superficies and the interior.

3. Also applicable to cases of influenza, poliomyelitis, infectious mononucleosis, mumps, acute cellulitis, erysipelas, acute lymphangitis, etc., which are attributive to simultaneous existence of sthenia – syndrome in the superficies and the interior after attack of exogenous wind – heat and retention of heat in the body.

Interpretation

Ledebouriellae, *Schizonepetae*, *Ephedrae*, *Zingiberis Recens* and *Menthae* serve to expel wind by sweating. *Rhei* and *Natrii Sulfas* eliminate the internal heat by purgation, and *Gardeniae* and *Talcum* clear away heat by diuresis. *Platycodi*, *Gypsum Fibrosum*, *Scutellariae* and *Forsythiae* can clear away heat from the lung and stomach. All the above drugs act together to eliminate heat from the upper and the lower part of the body, and treat both the superficies and the interior syndrome. *Angelicae Sinensis*, *Ligustici Chuanxiong* and *Paeoniae Alba* have the effects of expelling wind and nourishing blood, and *Atractylodis Macrocephalae* and *Glycyrrhizae* serve to strengthen the spleen and regulating the stomach; they cooperate each other to exert a diaphoretic effect without damaging the superficies, and exert a purgative effect without impairing the interior. In sum, this prescription involves the therapeutic principles of diaphoretic, heat – eliminating, purgative and tonifying simultaneously, aiming at clearing away the internal heat chiefly. The application of *Natrii Sulfas* and *Rhei* is for purging heat.

White Tiger Decoction
(Baihu tang)

Ingredients

Gypsum Fibrosum	30 g
Rhizoma Anemarrhenae	9 g
Radix Glycyrrhizae Praeparata	3 g
Semen Oryzae Nonglutionosae	9 g

All the above drugs are to be decocted in water for oral administration.

Efficacy

Clearing away heat and promoting the production of body fluid.

Indications

Yangming channel diseases marked by high fever, flushed face, polydipsia, profuse perspiration, aversion to heat and full forceful pulse. It can be modified to treat influenza, epidemic encephalitis B, epidemic cerebrospinal meningitis, pneumonia and septicemia indicating excessive heat syndrome in the qi system.

Cautions

It is not advisable for those whose exterior syndrome is not relieved, nor for those who have fever due to blood − deficiency or cold syndrome with pseudo − heat symptoms.

Decoction of Gypsum Fibrosum and Three Yellows
(Sanhuang shigao tang)

Ingredients

Gypsum Fibrosum (decocted first	30 g
Radix Scutellariae	10 g
Rhizoma Coptidis	10 g
Cortex Phellodendri	10 g
Fructus Gardeniae	10 g
Semen Sojae Praeparatum	10 g
Herba Ephedrae	3 g
Rhizoma Zingiberis Recens	3 pcs
Fructus Ziziphi Jujubae	2 pcs
Folium Camelliae Sinensis	6 g

Decoct the above ingredients in a right amount of water for oral administration.

Efficacy

Expelling the pathogens from both the interior and the superficies, purging fire and eliminating toxic materials; mainly for seasonal febrile diseases involving both the interior and superficies, which manifest as high fever, chilliness, anhidrosis, flushed cheeks, dryness of teeth and nose, extreme thirst, severe headache, irritability or even mania, red tongue with yellow fur, bounding and rapid or smooth and rapid pulse.

Indications

1. For cases with yang macules which are punctate or pieces and bright red in colour, accompanied with high fever, thirst, flushed cheeks, conjunctival congestion, red or crimson tongue with yellow fur, bounding and rapid pulse, which are attributive to stagnation of heat in the *yangming* channel involving *yingfen* and *xuefen*, use *Radix Rehmanniae* instead of *Ephedrae* and *Sojae Praepara-*

tum.

2. Also applicable to cases suffering from common cold, encephalitis B, typhoid fever and paratyphoid fever with high fever, which are attributive to attack of potent heat to both interior and the superficies; and to cases of epidemic hemorrhagic fever, typhus fever, which are attributive to the stagnation of heat in the *yangming* channel involving *yingfen* and *xuefen*.

3. Applicable to infections of skin and subcutaneous tissues acccompanied with high fever, irritability, extreme thirst, oliguria with reddish urine, red tongue with yellow fur, wiry and rapid pulse, which are attributive to retnetion of heat and toxic material in the superficies when the pathogens are potent and the healthy energy is still strong.

Interpretation

Gypsum Fibrosum can clear away the interior heat and acts as the chief drug of the prescription. *Ephedrae* and *Sojae Praeparatum* are applied to promote sweating and discharge the heat outside. The above three durgs used together can expel heat from both the interior and the superficies. Since there is a large amount of heat in the triple-jiao, *Scutellariae* is applied to clear away the heat in the upper-jiao. *Gardeniae* and *Camelliae Sinensis* can discharge the heat of triple-jiao from the urine. *Zingiberis* and *Ziziphi Jujubae* serve to regulate *ying* and *wei*.

Decoction of Ginseng for Nourishing Qi and Ying
(Renshen yang rong tang)

Ingredients

Radix Paeoniae Alba	15 g
Radix Rehmanniae Praeparata	15 g
Radix Codonopsis Pilosulae	10 g
Radix Astragali seu Hedysari	10 g
Rhizoma Atractylodis Macrocephalae	10 g

Commonly Used Recipes

Poria	10 g
Radix Angelicae Sinensis	10 g
Exocarpium Citri Grandis	6 g
Fructus Schisandrae	6 g
Radix Glycyrrhizae Praeparata	3 g
Cortex Cinnamomi	3 g
Radix Polygalae	3 g
Rhizoma Zingiberis Recens	3 pcs
Fructus Ziziphi Jujubae	3 pcs

Decoct the above ingredients in a right amount of water for oral administration.

Efficacy

Benefiting qi, tonifying blood, strengthening spleen and nourishing heart; mainly for consumptive diseases manifested by palpitation, amnesia, insomnia, dreaminess, tiredness, profuse sweating, poor appetite, shortness of breath, dyspnea upon exertion, pale tongue, sunken and weak pulse, which are attributive to insufficiency of qi and blood, and hypofunction of heart and spleen.

Indications

Applicable to cases of irregular (or delayed) menstruation with scanty pale discharge, sallow complexion, palpitation, dizziness, shortness of breath, fatigue, poor appetite, pale tongue, which are attributive to deficiency of liver - blood and spleen - qi and failure of releasing stagnated qi and controlling blood.

2. Also indicated for the late stage of pyogenic infection of skin when the acute inlammation subsides but the qi and blood are deficient, which manifest lesion with discharge of thin purulent fluid, dark greyish coloration but without granulation, and accompanied with lusterless complexion and pale tongue.

3. Also applicable to cases of pulmonary tuberculosis, rheumatic heart diseases, gastric ulcer, tuberculous abscess, carbuncle, phlebeurysma of the lower limbs, etc. which are attributive to deficiency of qi and blood.

Interpretation

The prescription is composed by omitting *Rhizoma Ligustici Chuanxiong* and adding *Astragali seu Hedysari*, *Cortex Cinnamomi*, *Citri Grandis*, *Schisandrae* and *Polygalae* to the *Decoction of Eight Ingredients for Tonifying Qi and Blood*. *Ligustici Chuanxiong* is omitted because the effect of activating blood circulation is not desired. The effect of tonifying blood and promoting blood production is obtained when *Astragali seu Hedysari* is used together with *Angelicae Sinensis*. *Cortex Cinnamomi* used together with *Zingiberis Recens*, *Ziziphi Jujubae* can accelerate the growth of qi and blood. *Polygalae* and *Schisandrae* adding to *Codonopsis Pilosulae* and *Astragali seu Hedysari* serve to benefit the heart — qi and tranquilizing. *Citri Grandis* is used for regulating qi and stomach to decrease the indigestibility of the tonics.

Ease Powder
(Xiao Yao San)

Ingredients

Radix bupleuri	15 g
Radix Angelicae Sinensis	15 g
Radix Paeoniae Alba	15 g
Poria	15 g
Rhizoma Atractylodis Macrocephalae	15 g
Rhizoma Zingiberis Recens Praeparata	3 g
Herba Menthae	3 g
Radix Glycyrrhizae Praeparata	6 g

Grind the above drugs except *ginger* and *peppermint* into powder take 6 to 9 grams each time with a decoction in small amount of roasted *ginger* and *peppermint*.

Efficacy

Soothing the liver disperse depressed qi, and invigorating the spleen to nourish the blood.

Indications

Stagnation of the liver – qi with deficiency of the blood marked by hypochondriac pain, headache, dizziness, bitter mouth, dry throat, mental weariness and poor appetite, or alternate attacks of chills and fever, or irregular menstruation, distension in the breast, light redness of the tongue, taut and feeble pulse.

Patients with chronic hepatitis, Pleuritis, chronic gastritis, neurosis, irregular menstruation marked by symptoms of stagnation of liver – qi with deficiency of the blood can be treated by the modified recipe.

Interpretation

Bupleurum root in the recipe soothes the liver to disperse the depressed qi. *Chinese yam* and *White peony root* nourish the blood and the liver. The joint use of the three drugs is able to treat the primary cause of stagnation of the liver – qi and deficiency of the blood. *Poria* and *Bighead atractylodes rhizome* strengthen the middle – jiao and reinforce the spleen so as to enrich the source of growth and development of the qi and blood. *Roasted ginger* regulates the stomach and warms the middle – jiao. *Peppermint* assists *Bupleurum root* in soothing the liver to disperse the depressed qi. *Prepared licorice root* can not only assist *Bighead atractylodes rhizome* and *Poria* in replenishing qi and invigorating the middle – warmer but also coordinate the effects of all the drugs in the recipe.

Modern researches have proved that the recipe has remarkable effects of nourishing the liver, tranquilizing the mind and relieving spasm. It is also effective in promoting digestion, coordinating uterine function, nourishing blood, strengthening the stomach and so on.

Decoction of Aneglicae Pubescentis and Taxilli
(Duhuo Jisheng Tang)

Ingredients

Radix Angelicae Pubescentis	10 g
Cortex Eucommiae	10 g
Radix Achyranthis Bidentatae	10 g
Radix Gentianae Macrophyllae	10 g
Poria	10 g
Radix Ledebouriellae	10 g
Radix Angelicae Sinensis	10 g
Radix Codonopsis Pilosulae	10 g
Radix Paeoniae Alba	10 g
Ramulus Taxilli	18 g
Radix Rehmanniae	18 g
Lignum Cinnamomi	1.5 g
Rhizoma Ligustici Chuanxiong	6 g
Herba Asari	3 g
Radix Glycyrrhizae	3 g

Decoct the above ingredients in a right amount of water for oral administration.

Efficacy

Expelling wind – dampness evil, relieving arthralgia, benefiting the liver and kidney, invigorating vital energy and blood; mainly for prolonged arthralgia of wind – cold – dampness type with hypofunction of liver and kidney and insufficiency of vital energy and blood, which is manifested as cold pain over the loin and joints, limited mobility and flaccidity of joints, or numbness, aversion to cold and desire for warmth, pale tongue with whitish fur, small and weak pulse.

Indications

1. Applicable to cases of stroke manifested by hemiplegia, numbness, spasm of limbs, pale tongue with whitish fur, small and weak pulse, which are attributive to deficiency of both the liver and the kidney, and attack of wind evil to the meridians.

2. Also applicable to cases of chronic rheumatic arthritis, rheumatic sciatica, lumbar strain, prolapse of lumbar intervertebral disc, etc., marked by cold pain over the loin and knees, which are attributive to prolonged bi-syndrome with deficiency of both the liver and the kidney and insufficiency of vital energy and blood.

Interpretation

Angelicae Pubescentis, *Ledebouriellae* and *Gentianae Macrophyllae* have the effects of expelling wind and dampness, *Asari* expels wind-cold evil from the yin-channel and eliminates wind-dampness evil from the muscles and tendons; the above three drugs used together exert an analgesic effect for rheumatism of wind-cold-dampness type evil and relieving pain. Prolonged rheumatism (attack of wind-cold-dampness evil) may aggravate the deficiency of liver and kidney, so *Ramulus Taxilli*, *Achyranthis Bidentatae* and *Eucommiae* are applied to tonify the liver and kidney, strengthen the tendons and bones, *Codonopsis Pilosulae*, *Poria*, *Glycyrrhizae* to invigorate healthy energy, and *Rehmanniae*, *Angelicae Sinensis* and *Paeoniae Alba* to nourish blood and activate blood circulation. Moreover, *Ligustici Chuanxiong* and *Lignum Cinnamomi* are added to warm and dredge the vessels and expel wind evil. In sum, the prescription serves as both symptomatic and causative therapy for arthralgia by supplementing vital energy and blood, invigorating liver and kidney, and eliminating wind.

Decoction for Pus Drainage and Relieving Pain
(Tuoli ding tong tang)

Ingredients

Radix Rehmanniae Praeparata	18 g
Radix Angelicae Sinensis	12 g
Radix Paeoniae Alba	12 g
Rhizoma Ligustici Chuanxiong	8 g
Pericarpium Papaveris	8 g
Cortex Cinnamomi	3 g
Olibanum	3 g
Myrrhae	3 g

Decoct the above ingredients in a right amount of water for oral administration.

Efficacy

Nourishing blood, promoting granulation, eliminating blood stasis and relieving pain; mainly for unhealed carbuncle after rupture with thin purulent bloody discharge, severe pain, poor granulation, pale tongue, small and rapid pulse.

Indications

1. Applicable to cases of dysmenorrhea with oligomenorrhea and darkish discharge, fatigue, pale or darkish tongue, sunken and small, unsmooth pulse, which are attributive to deficiency and stagnation of blood.

2. Also applicable to cases of thromboangiitis obliterans, chronic ulcer of lower extremity and tuberculosis of cervical lymph nodes with unhealed wound and poor granulation and case of endometriosis, endometritis, hysteromyoma and vegetative neurosis marked by dysmenorrhe, which are attributive to deficiency and stagnation of blood.

Interpretation

Olibanum and *Myrrhae* promote blood circulation and remove blood stasis to relieve pain. *Rehmanniae Praeparata*, *Angelicae Sinensis*, *paeoniae Alba* and *Ligustici Chuanxiong* are used for nourishing blood to promote granulation and help the first two drugs to promote blood circulation and relieve pain. A small dosage of *Cinnamomi* combined with *Rehmannaie Praeparata* and *Angelicae Sinensis* has the effects of activating the blood and vital qi circulation and promoting granulation. *Pericarpium Papaveris* exerts a prompt astringent and analgesic effect.

Xiaojin Pellet
(Xiao jin dan)

Ingredients

Resina Liquidambaris	3 g
Radix Aconiti Kusnezoffii	6 g
Olibanum	6 g
Myrrha	6 g
Faeces Trogropterori	10 g
Radix Angelicae Sinensis	10 g
Lumbricus	10 g
Carbonized Chinese ink	1 g

The above drugs are ground into powder and prepared as pellets, taken with rice wine.

Efficacy

Eliminating cold, expelling phlegm, removing blood stasis and reducing swelling; mainly for multiple abscesses, subcutaneous nodules, scrofula, and osteomyelitis with local pain and swelling, which are attributive to retention of phlegm – dampness evil in the meridians.

Indications

1. Applcable to cases of stomachache with tenderness, or hematemesis with purplish-dark discharge, darkish tongue with white and smooth fur, unsmooth pulse, which are attributive to stagnation of blood and phlegm.

2. Also applicable to cases of cold abscess, tuberculous lymphadenitis, tuberculosis of joints and chronic osteomyelitis attributive to the stagnation of cold-phlegm and dampness; also to cases of gastric cancer and breast carcinoma attribvutive to the stagnation of blood and phlegm.

Interpretation

Aconit Kusnezoffii has the effects of eliminating cold and dampness, dredging the passage of meridians, reducing swelling and alleviating pain. *Momordicae and Resina Liquidambaris* serve to reduce swelling and alleviate pain. *Moschus* can reopen the meridians, remove blood stasis and relieve swelling. The above four drugs serve as the principal drugs in the prescription. *Lumbricus* used together with *Aconiti Kusnezoffii* can eliminate phlegm and cold, dredge the passage of meridians and activate yang. *Carbonized Chinese ink* used together with *Moschus* can eliminate dampness, remove blood stasis and reduce swelling. *Olibanum, Myrrha, Faeces Trogopterori* and *rice wine* can activate blood circulation, reduce swelling and alleviate pain. *Angelicae Sinensis* is applied for nourishing blod, so that the healthy qi will not be impaired when blood stasis is removed by other drugs. It also enhances the effect of *Aconiti Kusnezoffii*.

Decoction for Warming Yang
(Yang he tang)

Ingredients

Radix Rehmanniae Praeparata	30 g
Cortex Cinnamomi	3 g
Herba Ephedrae	2 g

Colla Cornus Cervi	9 g
Semen Sinapis Albae	6 g
Rhizoma Zingiberis Praeparata	2 g
Radix Glycyrrhizae	3 g

Decoct the above ingredients in a right amount of water for oral administration.

Efficacy

Warming yang, tonifying blood, expelling cold and dispersing stagnation; mainly for yin type carbuncle, bone carbuncle, multiple abscesses and arthroncus of knee joint, attributive to deficiency of blood and stagnation of cold evil, manifested by local and not well - demarcated swelling, no change of color and temperature, no pain or just mild aching, pale tongue with whitish and smooth fur, sunken and slow pulse.

Indications

1. For cases of yin type carbuncle with pale tongue, floating and large pulse, complicated by deficiency of vital qi, add raw *Radix Astragali seu Hedysari* to benefit vital qi and promot pus drainage.

2. Applicable to cases of dyspneic cough with profuse and thin sputum, which are attributive to hypofunction of both lung and kidney with retention of dampness - phlegm, in this case the prescription is used for warming and invigorating the lung and kidney, eliminating sputum and relieving dyspnea. It may also be applied for cases of bi - syndrome and dysmenorrhea attributive to blood deficiency and cold - stagnation, and serves to warm yang, tonify blood, expel cold evil and arrest pain in this case.

3. Also applicable to cases of deep abscess, bone tuberculosis, chronic osteomyelitis, rheumatic arthritis, tuberculosis of knee joint, etc. which are attributive to blood - deficiency and cold - stagnation.

Interpretation

Rehmanniae Praeparata has the effcts of warming and tonifying ying – blood and inhibiting diaphoretic effect of *Ephedrae*, so that the latter preserves the action of warming the striae. *Colla Cornus Cervi* can produce essence substance, nourish bone marrow and blood, and support yang. It also inhibits the "dispersing" effect of *Cinnamomi* and *Zingiberis* and renders them just for warming and dredging the channels, and removing the stagnation of cold and phlegm. In turn, *Cinnamomi* and *Zingiberis* render *Rehmanniae Praeparata* and *Colla Cornus Cervi* exerting tonic effect but not greasy. *Ephedrae* distributes to the superficis, while *Rehmanniae Praeparata* to the interior. Two drugs help each other to warm and dredgethe striae and channels. *Sinapis Albae* serve to eliminate phlegm and disperse the stagnation of evil. *Glycyrrhizae* is used rawly just for detoxification. In summary, this prescription does not stress on the elimination of toxic material for the treatment of yin type carbuncle. It composed of drugs for warming yang, nourishing blood, dispersing cold and dredging stagnation of evil, thus embodies the therapeutic principle that the root cause of the disease must be aimed at.

Decoction of Persicae for Purgation
(Taohe chengqi tang)

Ingredients

Semen Persicae	12 g
Radix et Rhizoma Rhei	12 g
Ramulus Cinnamomi	10 g
Radix Glycyrrhizae Praeparata	6 g
Natrii Sulfas	6 g

Decoct the above ingredients in a right amount of water for oral administration.

Efficacy

Eliminating blood stasis and purging heat evil; mainly for blood – stagnation syndrome due to accumulation of blood stasis and heat evil in the lower jiao, which is manifested by distending pain over the lower abdomen, irritability, sunken and solid pulse.

Indications

1. For cases of preceded menstrual cycle, amenorrhea, metrorrhagia, etc., attributive to combination of blood stasis and heat evil in the lower jiao, omit *Glycyrrhizae* from the prescription and add *Radix Angelicae Sinensis* to regulate meenstruation, activate blood circulation, eliminate blood stasis and stop bleeding.
2. For cases of abdominal pain after operation due to blood stasis, or trauma (especially the early stage of fracture of thoracic or lumbar vertebrae), which are attributive to combination of blood stasis and heat evil, omit *Glycyrrhizae* and add *Radix Cyathulae* to activate blood circulation and eliminate blood stasis, and let the blood flowing downwards.
3. Applicable to cases of hematemesis, headache, congestion of conjunctiva, which are attributive to upward attack of blood stasis and heat evil.
4. Also applicable to cases of intestinal obstruction, pelvic cellulitis, appendicitis, etc. with abdominal pain, or cases of retention of placenta, dysfunctional uterine bleeding, etc. with headache or bleeding from the gum, which are attributive to combination or upward attack of blood stasis and heat evil.

Major Decoction for Purging Down Digestive Qi
(Da chengqi tang)

Ingredients

Radix et Rhizoma Rhei	12 g
Cortex Magnoliae Officinalis	15 g

Fructus Aurantii Immaturus	12 g
Natrii Sulfas	9 g

Decoct the above ingredients in a right amount of water for oral administration.

Efficacy

Expelling pathogenic heat and loosening the bowel, promoting the circulation of qi to purge accumulation in the bowels.

Indications

1. Excessive – heat syndrome of *yangming – fu* organ, manifested by constipation, frequent wind through the anus, feeling of fullness in the abdomen, abdominal pain with tenderness and guarding, tidal fever, delirium, polyhidrosis of hands and feet, prickled tongue with yellow dry fur or dry black tongue coating with fissures, deep and forceful pulse.
2. Syndrome of fecal impaction due to heat with watery discharge, manifested by watery discharge of terribly foul odor accompnaied by abdominal distension and pain with tenderness and guarding, dry mouth and tongue, smooth and forceful pulse.
3. Cold limbs due to excess of heat, convulsion, mania and other symptoms belonging to excess syndrome of interior heat.

Equally, this recipe can be modified to deal with infectious or non – infectious febrile diseasesin their climax marked by accumulation of heat type, and in the treatment of paralytic, simple and obliterative intestinal obstructions.

Interpretation

Rhei has the purgative effect and eliminating heat, but cannot induce an immediate purgation since it only promotes the peristalsis of large intestine and cannot soften the dry feces. While *Natrii Sulfas* can creat a hypertonic condition in the large intestine and retain enough amount of water to softne the dry feces. hence the two drugs used together may give an immediate purgation. Moreover,

Magnoliae Officinalis and *Aurantii Immaturus* have the effects of promoting vital qi circulation and relieving distension in the abdomen, so as to regulate the function of the gastrointestine, and enhance the effect of *Rhei* and *Natrii Sulfas*.

Major Decoction of Bupleurum
(Da chaihu tang)

Ingredients

Radix Bupleuri	15 g
Radix Scutellariae	9 g
Radix Paeoniae Alba	9 g
Rhizoma Pinelliae	9 g
Fructus Aurantii Immaturus Praeparata	9 g
Radix et Rhizoma Rhei	6 g
Rhizoma Zingiberis Recens	15 g
Fructus Ziziphi Jujubae	5 pcs

Decoct the above ingredients in a right amount of water for oral administration.

Efficacy

Treating *shaoyang* disease by mediation and purging away internal stasis of heat.

Indications

Shaoyang and *yangming* diseases complex marked by alternate attacks of chills and fever, fullness and oppression in the chest, hypochondriac discomfort, frequent vomiting, mental depression and dysphoria, epigastric fullness and pain or epigastric rigidity, constipation or diarrhea due to interior cold and exterior heat, yellow tongue fur, stringy and forceful pulse.

Patients with acute cholecystitis, cholelithiasis, acute pancreatitis and infection of abdominal activity marked by the above-mentioned symptoms can be treated by the modified recipe.

Pill of Stephaniae Tetrandrae, Zanthoxyli, Lepidii seu Descurainiae and Rhei
(Ji jiao li huang wan)

Ingredients

Radix Stephaniae Tetrandrae	10 g
Semen Zanthoxyli	10 g
Semen Lepidii seu Descurainiae	10 g
Radix et Rhizoma Rhei	6 g

Decoct the above ingredients in a right amount of water for oral administration.

Efficacy

Eliminating the retained fluid and discharging the evils from the lower part; mainly for phlegm-retention syndrome manifested by abdominal fullness, loose stools, dry mouth and tongue, sunken and wiry pulse, which is attributive to retention of fluid in the intestines when the healthy energy is still strong and the evil is hyperactive.

Indications

1. Applicable to cases of dyspneic cough accompanied by feeling of fullness over the chest, inability to lie flat, profuse expectoration, constipation, oliguria, yellow and greasy fur, wiry and smooth pulse, which are attributive to retention of fluid in the thorax.
2. Also inidcated for cases of dysuria accompanied with dyspnea, constipation, floating and smooth pulse, which are attributive to stagnation of phlegm-

heat in the lung, and adverse rising of qi.

3. Also applicable to cases of cirrhosis of liver, chronic nephritis, idiopathic edema, tuberculous pleurisy, lung cancer with pleuralmetastasis, acute glomerular nephritis, urinary infection, etc. which are attributive to fluid or phlegm retention.

Powder of Bupleuri for Dispersing the Depressed Liver – Qi (Chaihu shugan san)

Ingredients

Radix Bupleuri	10 g
Fructus Aurantii	10 g
Rhizoma Ligustici Chuanxiong	10 g
Exocarpium Citri Grandis	10 g
Rhizoma Cyperi	10 g
Radix Paeoniae Alba	15 g
Radix Glycyrrhizae Praeparata	6 g

Decoct the above ingredients in a right amount of water for oral administration.

Efficacy

Dispersing the stagnated liver – qi, regulating vital qi, activating blood circulation and relieving pain; mainly for ceses due to stagantion of liver – qi and vital qi manifested by fullness of breast, hypochondriac pain, or dysmenorrhea, or stomachache, and for cases due to stagnation of liver and gallbladder heat manifested by alternating episodes of chills and fever.

Indications

1. This prescription and *Powder for Treating Yang Exhaustion* both have the similar action and indication, but the former, owning to the action of *Bupleuri*,

ahs a stronger effect on dispersing the stagnated liver-qi, regulating the vital qi and adtivating blood circulation. It is frequently applied for the cases of menoxenia or distending pain of the breast.

2. For cases with distending pain of the breast, add *Radix Salviae Miltiorrhizae* and *Fructus Hordei Germinatus* (30 g) to disperse the stagnated liver-qi and promote blood circulation; for cases with alternating epidsodes cf chills and fever, omit *Ligustici Chuanxiong* and add *Radix Scutellariae* and *Herba Artemisiae Annuae* to clear away the gallbladder heat.

3. Also applicable to cases of pleurisy, cholecystitis, mastitis, hyperplasia of mammary gland, etc., which are attributive to stagnation of liver-qi and vital qi.

Decoction of Gentianae for Purging Liver-Fire
(Longdan xie gan tang)

Ingredients

Herba Gentianae	6 g
Radix Bupleuri	6 g
Radix Glycyrrhizae	6 g
Rhizoma Alismatis	10 g
Semen Plantaginis	10 g
Caulis Akebiae	10 g
Radix Rehmanniae	10 g
Fructus Gardeniae	10 g
Radix Scutellariae	10 g
Radix Angelicae Sinensis	3 g

Decoct the above ingredients in a right amount of water for oral administration.

Efficacy

Purging the sthenia fire of liver and gallbladder, clearing away the dampness

— heat evil from triple jiao; mainly for cases with flaming up of sthenia fire in the liver and gallbladder, manifested by headache, hypochondriac pain, bitter taste in the mouth, congestion of the conjunctiva and deafness, and for cases with downward attack of dampness — heat from the liver and gallbladder, manifested by stranguria with turbid urine, pruritus vulvae and leukorrhagia.

Indications

1. For cases of jaundice attributive to dampness — heat attacking the liver and gallbladder, omit *Glycyrrhizae* and *Rehmanniae* and add *Herba Artemisiae Scopariae* and *Radix et Rhizoma Rhei* to eliminate the heat evil through urination and defecation.

2. For cases of leukorrhagia, with yellow or red and white, thick, foul discharge, red tongue with yellowish and greasy fur, smooth and rapid pulse, which are attributive to downward attack of dampness — heat from the liver meridian, omit *Glycyrrhizae* and use *Cortex Phellodendri* instead of *Scutellariae*.

3. Also applicable to cases of acute conjunctivitis, acute otitis media, furuncle of the vestibulum nasi and external auditory canal, hypertension which are attributive to flaming up of sthenia fire in the liver and gallbladder; to cases of icteric hepatitis, cholecystitis, herpes zoster which are attributive to retention of dampness — heat evil in the liver and gallbladder; to cases of urinary infection, pelvic inflammation, prostatitis, which are attributive to downward attack of dampness — heat evil from the liver and gallbladder.

Pulse — Activating Powder
(Sheng mai san)

Ingredients

Radix Ginseng	10 g
Radix Ophiopogonis	15 g
Fructus Schisandrae	6 g

Decoct the above ingredients in a right amount of water for oral administration.

Efficacy

Supplementing qi, promoting the production of body fluid, astringing yin-fluid and arresting sweat.

Indications

Syndrome of impairment of both qi and yin manifested by general debility, shortness of breath, disinclination to talk, thirst with profuse sweat, dry tongue and throat, deficient and weak pulse, or impairment of the lung due to chronic cough, dry cough with shortness of breath, spontaneous perspiration or palpitation, and faint pulse with tendency to exhaustion.

The recipe can be modified to deal with dehydrant shock caused by heat stroke, bleeding, severe vomiting or diarrhea, dramatic injury, scald; or syndrome of impairment of both qi and yin as seen in cases at recovery stage of febrile diseases or at postoperation, or in cases with chronic disorders; or syndrome of deficiency of both qi and yin as seen in such cases as tuberculosis, chronic bronchitis, bronchiectasis, etc..

Cautions

Since it has an astringing effect, it is neither fit for patients whose exopathogen has not been dispelled, nor for those with hyperactivity of heat due to summer-heat diseases, but without impairment of qi and body fluid.

Decoction for Rashes Subsidence
(Hua ban tang)

Ingredients

Gypsum Fibrosum   30 g

Rhizoma Anemarrhenae	12 g
Radix Scrophulariae	10 g
Radix Glycyrrhizae	6 g
Cornu Rhinocerotis	6 g
Semen Oryzae Sativae	20 g

Decoct the above ingredients in a right amount of water for oral administration.

Efficacy

Clearing away heat evil and toxic material, cooling blood and letting tghe rashes subsided; mainly for cases attributive to involvement of qifen and xuefen by severe heat and extravasation of blood - heat, which are manifested by high fever, dark - red rashes, dry mouth, restlessness, or even unconsciousness and delinum, red tongue with yellow fur.

Indications

1. This prescription is applied for cases due to involvement of xuefen by severe heat in qifen, or involvement of both xuefen and qifen by severe heat.

2. Applicable to cases attributive to attack of the stomach by liver - fire with damage of the stomach vessels, which are manifested by hematemesis, irritability, red tongue with yellow fur, wiry and rapid pulse.

3. For cases attributive to hyperactivity of stomach - fire with involvement of blood, which are manifested by tooth bleeding, gingivitis, headache, foul breath, red tongue with yellow fur, bounding and rapid pulse, add ***Radix Cyathulae*** to let the fire running downward.

4. Also applicable to cses of typnus, erysipelas, epidemic meningitis, septicemia, etc. with fever and skin rashes attributive to involvement of qifen and xuefen by severe heat, or cases of esophageal varicosis with hematemesis attributive to attack of the stomach by liver - fire, or cases of periodontal diseases, necrotizing ulcerative gingivitis with tooth bleeding attributive to hyperactivity of stomach - fire.

Decoction of Restoration
(Fuyuan huoxue tang)

Ingredients

Radix Bupleuri	10 g
Radix Trichosanthis	10 g
Radix Angelicae Sinensis	10 g
Squama Manitis Praeparata	10 g
Radix et Rhizoma Rhei	10 g
Semen Persicae	10 g
Flos Carthami	6 g
Radix Glycyrrhizae	3 g
wine	q.s.

Decoct the above ingredients in a right amount of water for oral administration.

Efficacy

Activating blood circulation, removing blood stasis, dispersing the depressed liver − qi and dredging the passage of meridians; mainly for cases of swelling and pain over the chest and hypochondrium due to trauma.

Indications

1. This is a commonly − used prescription for traumata of chest and hypochondrium with swelling, pain and ecchymoses. For injury of the upper limbs, add *Ramulus Cinnamomi*; for that of the lower limbs, add *Radix Achyranthis Bidentatae*.

2. Also applicable to cases with chest intercostal neuralgia and costal chondritis which are attributive to retention of blood stasis.

Decoction for Severe Phlegm – Heat Syndrome in the Chest
(Da xian xiong tang)

Ingredients

Radix et Rhizoma Rhei	12 g
Natrii Sulfas	10 g
Radix Euphorbiae Kansui (powder, not for decocting)	1.5 g

Decoct the above ingredients in a right amount of water for oral administration.

Efficacy

Purging, eliminating water retention, relieving the accumulation of heat evil; mainly for syndrome attributive to evil accumulating in the thorax, manifested by severe pain and tenderness over the upper abdomen, fever, constipation, sunken and tense pulse, etc..

Indications

1. This prescription is applied for a critical case and should be used as early as possible. Diarrhea usually occurs half an hour after the decoction is taken. One dose may be repeated if diarrhea does not occur after one hour. Overdosage should be prohibited, otherwise the healthy qi may be impaired.

2. Also applicable to cases of acute pancreatitis edematous type, and acute cholecystitis, which are attributive to simultaneous attack of water and heat evil.

Decoction for Soothing the Intestine
(Chang ning tang)

Ingredients

Radix Angelicae Sinensis	15 g

Radix Rehmanniae Praeparata	15 g
Radix Codonopsis Pilosulae	10 g
Radix Ophiopogonis	10 g
Colla Corii Asini	10 g
Rhizoma Dioscoreae	10 g
Radix Dipsaci	10 g
Radix Glycyrrhizae	3 g
Cortex Cinnamomi	1 g

Decoct the above ingredients in a right amount of water for oral administration.

Efficacy

Nourishing blood and benefiting vital qi; mainly for cases of postpartum anemia with dull aching over the lower abdomen which can be relieved by pressing, discharge of scanty thin lochia, dizziness, tinnitus, palpitation, amnesia, pale complexion, constipation, pale tongue, small and weak pulse.

Indications

1. Applicable to cases of metrorrhagia with profuse thin and pale discharge, spiritlessness, dizziness, tinnitus, lumbago, weakness of knees, darkish complexion, pale tongue, sunken and small, weak pulse, which are attributive to impairment of liver and kidney and deficiency of blood and vital qi.

2. Also indicated for cases of ecthyma accompanied with pale tongue, small and rapid pulse, which are attributive to deficiency of blood and vital qi.

3. Also applicable to cases of chronic pelvic inflammation, hypofunction of anterior pituitary, chronic hypoadrenocorticism, dysfunctional uterine bleeding, phlebeurysma of lower limbs, chronic osteomyelitis, which are attributive to deficiency of blood and vital qi.

Decoction of Angelicae Sinensis for Analgesic
(Danggui niantong tang)

Ingredients

Rhizoma seu Radix Notopterygii	10 g
Herba Artemisiae Scopariae	10 g
Radix Ledebouriellae	10 g
Polyporus Umbellatus	10 g
Radix Puerariae	10 g
Rhizoma Atractylodis	10 g
Radix Angelicae Sinensis	12 g
Rhizoma Atractylodis Macrocephalae	12 g
Radix Scutellariae	8 g
Rhizoma Anemarrhenae	8 g
Rhizoma Alismatis	6 g
Rhizoma Cimicifugae	6 g
Radix Codonopsis Pilosulae	6 g
Radix Sophorae Flavescentis	6 g
Radix Glycyrrhizae Praeparata	3 g

Decoct the above ingredients in a right amount of water for oral administration.

Efficacy

Drying dampness, clearing away heat, activating blood circulation and expelling wind, mainly for cases attributive to attack of dampness and heat, which manifest swelling and pain of the joints, fever, aversion to wind, feeling of oppression over the chest, yellow and greasy fur on the tongue, soft and floating, slow or smooth and rapid pulse.

Indications

1. For cases of wet beriberi with oliguira, yellow and greasy fur on the

tongue, soft and floating, slow pulse, which are attributive to retention of dampness — heat in the meridians and stagnation of vital energy and blood, increase the dosage of *Atractylodis* and decrease the dose of *Scutellariae* and *Anemarrhenae*.

2. Also indicated for cases attributive to retention of dampness and toxic material in the muscles and skin, when manifest pyogenic infection of skin, accompanied with fever, thirst, yellow and greasy fur on tongue, soft and floating, slow pulse.

3. Also applicable to cases of rheumatic arthritis, periomarthritis, multiple neuritis, etc. which are attributive to retention of dampness — heat in the meridians; and to cases of impetigo, folliculitis, paronychia, etc. attributive to retention of dampness and toxic material in the muscles and skin.

Decoction of Angelicae Sinensis for Warming Cold Limbs
(Danggui sini tang)

Ingredients

Radix Angelicae Sinensis	10 g
Ramulus Cinnamomi	10 g
Radix Paeoniae Alba	12 g
Herba Asari	6 g
Radix Glycyrrhizae Praeparata	6 g
Caulis Akebiae	6 g
Fructus Ziziphi Jujubae	6 pcs

Decoct the above ingredients in a right amount of water for oral administration.

Efficacy

Warming the channel, expelling cold evil, nourishing blood and dredging the passage of channels; mainly for cases due to deficiency of blood, attack of cold evil and impediment of blood circulation, which are manifested by cold limbs, indistinct pulse, pale tongue with whitish fur.

Indications

1. For cases of dysmenorrhea attributive to deficiency of blood and presence of cold evil, omit *Akebiae* and add *Radix Rehmanniae Praeparata* to nourish the blood and regulate menstruation.

2. For cases with cold colic testalgia referring to the lower abdomen, sunken and wiry pulse, add *Fructus Foeniculi* to warm the liver and regulate vital energy.

4. Also aplicable to cases with cold limbs or abdominal pain occurring in thromboangiitis, *Raynaud*'s disease, acrocyanosis, chilblain, indirect inguinal hernia, dysmenorrhea, etc., which are attributive to blood deficiency and affection of cold evil.

Bolus for Severe Endogenous Wind – Syndrome
(Da Ding Feng Zhu)

INGREDIENTS

Radix Paeoniae Alba	18 g
Radix Rehmanniae	18 g
Colla Corii Asini	10 g
Radix Ophiopogonis	10 g
Plastrum Testudinis	12 g
Concha Ostreae	12 g
Carapax Trionycis	12 g
Semen Sesami	6 g
Fructus Schisandrae	6 g
Radix Glycyrrhizae Praeparata	3 g
Fresh egg yolk	1

EFFICACY

Nourishing yin and calming wind, mainly for cases of clonic convulsion attributive to damge of true-yin by heat and hyperactivity of liver-wind, which are accompanied with listlessness, crimson and uncoated tongue, small and weak pulse.

INDICATIONS

1. Indicated for cases attributive to deficiency of liver-yin and kidney-yin and upward attack of liver-yang, which are manifested as dizziness aggravated by over strain or anger, soreness of the loin and knees, insomnia and dreaminess, nocturnal emission, fatigue, bright red tongue, small and rapid pulse.

2. Also applicable to cases of encephalitis B, epidemic meningitis, poliomyelitis and chorea, marked by convulsion, which are attributive to damage of true-yin by heat and hyperactivity of liver-wind.

INTERPRETATION

Egg yolk and Colla Corii Asini are applied to nourish yin-fluid, supplement the exhausted true-yin and calm liver-wind. Rehmanniae, Sesami, Ophiopogonis and Paeoniae Alba serve to nourish yin and blood, soothe the liver and calm wind. Plastrum Testudinis, Concha Ostreae and Carapax Trionycis can invigorate kidney-yin and suppress hyperactive liver-yang.

Radix Glycyrrhizae Praeparata and Fructus Schisandrae are helpful for yin nourishing and wind calming.

Bolus of Arisaematis
(Tiannanxing Wan)

INGREDIENTS

Arisaema cum Bile	10 g
Radix Angelicae Dahuriacae	10 g
Radix Ledebouriellae	10 g
Rhizoma et Radix Notopterygii	10 g
Radix Angelicae Pubescentis	10 g
Rhizoma Ligustici Chuanxiong	10 g
Rhizoma Gastrodiae	10 g
Radix Paeoniae Alba	10 g
Bombyx Batryticatus	10 g
Herba Ephedrae	6 g
Radix Platycodi	6 g
Herba Asari	6 g
Radix Glycyrrhizae Praeparata	6 g
Rhizoma Zingiberis	6 g
Borneolum Syntheticum	3 g
Moschus	0.6 g

Administration: All the above ingredients are to be prepared with honey as boluses.

EFFICACY

Expelling wind evil and phlegm, waking up the patient and dredging the meridians; mainly for cases of stroke attributed to accumulation of wind-phlegm evil in the interior, which are manifested as numbness of limbs, hemiplegia, aphasia, whitish and greasy fur on the tongue, floating and smooth pulse.

INDICATIONS

1. Applicable to cases with swelling pain and immobility of joints, numbness of skin and muscle, whitish and greasy fur on the tongue, smooth pulse, which are attributed to artharalgia of wind – cold – dampness type.
2. Also applicable to cases of cerebral accidents, chronic rheumatic arthritis, sciatica, cervical vertebra syndrome, etc. manifested as hemiplegia, or arthralgia, or numbness of limbs, which are attributed to accumulation of wind – phlegm evil in the interior or arthralgia of wind – cold – dampness type.

INTERPRETATION

Arisaema cum Bile has a potent effect of expelling wind – phlegm evil and dredging the meridians, and acts as the chief drugs in the prescription. Bombyx Batryticatus enhances the effect of Arisaema cum Bile; Ledebouriellae, Notopterygii, Angelicae Pubescentis, Angelicae Dahuricae and Herba Menthae are helpful to expel wind evil and eliminate the dampness evil. Since phlegm – dampness evil is of yin nature, so Zingiberis and Asari are applied to warm the meridians and expel cold evil, and also help Arisaema cum Bile to dry the dampness and eliminate phlegm, so that the mobility of the extremities will be restored. Borneolum Syntheticum and Moschus have the effect of dredging the meridians, and are helpful to relieve aphasia. Gastrodiae, Glycyrrhizae Praeparata, Ligustici Chuanxiong and Paeoniae Alba have the effects of regulating vital energy and blood, subduing endogenous wind evil and relieving convulsion.

图书在版编目(CIP)数据

中医治疗耳鼻喉科疾病:英文版/侯景伦主编;
赵昕,李国华编 - 北京:学苑出版社,1997.6
ISBN7 - 5077 - 1362 - 8

Ⅰ.中… Ⅱ.①侯… ②赵… ③李… Ⅲ.①耳鼻咽喉病 - 中医治疗法 - 英文 Ⅳ.R276.1

中国版本图书馆 CIP 数据核字(97)第 10967 号

中医治疗耳鼻喉科疾病

主编 侯景伦

编委 赵 昕 李国华

学苑出版社出版
(中国北京万寿路西街 11 号)
邮政编码 100036
北京大兴沙窝店印刷厂印刷
中国国际图书贸易总公司发行
(中国北京车公庄西路 35 号)
北京邮政信箱第 399 号 邮政编码 100044
英文版 16 开本
1997 年 6 月第 1 版第 1 次印刷
ISBN7 - 5077 - 1362 - 8/R·272

08900
14 - E - 3171P